Words from ou

"Joshua Freitas has channeled his considerable energy and passion toward educating the public about dementia and how our society can better understand this condition. This book is a wonderful tool for bringing compassion, as well as better and more effective practices to dementia treatment."
Laurie Ann Cozad, Ph.D., Professor at Lesley University

"Joshua Freitas is one of those individuals who you come across only once in a lifetime and who leaves an indelible mark on the world around them. Joshua has an incredible passion for exploring ideas and possibilities for improving the lives of memory-impaired individuals and their families. He implements his ideas in ways that make a significant and meaningful difference for all."
Barbara Lenihan, MS, RN, CNS, CDP

"Watching Joshua interact with memory-impaired residents is heartwarming, inspiring, and educational. His compassion, education, and commitment to excellent care are exceptional. His techniques continually create positive relationships. Working with Joshua has been an invaluable experience. I have benefitted greatly from adopting his techniques into my own day-to-day practice as an RN."
Matt Sakakeeny, RN

"I may be old, but Joshua keeps me going. I have known Joshua for about two years. Ever since I was diagnosed with Alzheimer's, he has made himself available to help me and my family. He has shown me that my diagnosis is not the end of my life, and in some ways, it is simply the beginning of a new life. His advice has freed me from worrying about what others will think and helped me to just do what makes me happy."
Anonymous

The Dementia Concept:

Understand, Connect, Engage

Joshua J. Freitas

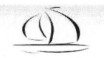

Blue Sail Publications, Inc.
Massachusetts, USA

Cover design: Judith Krimski, Krimski Design & Illustration

Neither the publisher nor the author is engaged in rendering professional advice or services to the individual reader. The ideas, procedures, and suggestions in this book are not intended as a substitute for consulting with a physician. All matters regarding health require medical supervision. Neither the author nor the publisher shall be liable or responsible for any loss or damage allegedly arising from any information or suggestion in this book. The reader should regularly consult a medical or behavioral professional in matters relating to his/her health, treatment, and care planning, particularly with respect to any symptoms that may require diagnosis or medical attention.

The Dementia Concept uses research-inspired philosophies, which may not work for everyone. Caring for, or working with persons who are living with dementia is by its nature potentially dangerous. Suggested approaches and techniques should be avoided if they put you or the person in your care at any harm or risk.

While the author has made every effort to provide accurate telephone numbers and Internet addresses at the time of publication, neither the publisher nor the author assumes any responsibility for errors or changes that occur after publication. Further, the publisher does not have any control over and does not assume any responsibility for author or third-party websites or their content. All recommendations are for informational purposes only, and neither the author nor the publisher are responsible for any consequences that may occur if readers follow the advice.

The Dementia Concept is a collection of non-pharmacological, person-centric discoveries and approaches to dementia care. In references to specific resident examples, names have been changed to respect privacy.

PUBLISHER'S NOTE

Joshua J. Freitas, CAEd, CADDCT, CDP, is an award-winning memory care program developer and researcher. He is focused on pushing the dementia care industry forward with the cutting-edge research and training philosophy described in this book. He holds five certifications related to dementia care and has studied at some of the world's most renowned colleges and universities, including Lesley University, Harvard University, and Berklee College of Music.

Joshua J. Frietas developed these dementia and memory care principles based on his training and a decade of fieldwork in private and professional memory care settings.

Angela Simonelli, CAC, is the Executive Editor of Blue Sail Publications, Inc., and the Supportive Writer and Developmental Editor of this book.

DEDICATION

I dedicate this book to a man named Alan who changed my life. He was the kind of friend who seemed more like family, and he was an important mentor to me because of his tremendous, positive insights about hope and life. When I began working with Alan, he was in the early stages of his dementia diagnosis. At that time, most people could not yet tell that he was suffering from any form of memory impairment. When his condition declined, Alan could barely speak and he lost the ability to walk. He never lost his sense of humor or his warm smile, which I'll never forget. He smiled every time I talked to him until his final days.

My friendship with Alan taught me patience and showed me that I could improve the lives of others by treating them with respect and understanding. The positivity and resilience of people like Alan have inspired me to dedicate my life to improving the quality of dementia care. It's important to remember that every person is a complex, vibrant, unique individual who deserves genuine connection and engagement with life. Dementia caregivers have a profound opportunity to facilitate and improve that connection and engagement.

Alan once told me, "Each day is new. Each day is my reward." What an inspiring and hopeful insight to come from a man who, by some estimations, had lost so much. Every day in my practice, I remember his grateful attitude. It reassures me of the fact that the person I am working with is still there, even if some of their functional abilities have been diminished.

Alan, you were a great man even when you struggled. You taught me so much. I will never forget you. This book is for you.

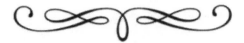

*"Though my mind may be going, I am still here.
I think; I live; I enjoy the company of those around me.
My only request is that everyone would stop asking if
I am okay. I am fine. I may even be better than fine
at this point in my life.*

*If I had to give advice to someone who has been
diagnosed with dementia, it would be to keep a sense
of humor. Life is too short to get caught up on
everything. If you get sick, you get sick, and that is that.
You just have to make the best of it."*

Alan Hochberg

CONTENTS

PART 3: ENGAGE

FOREWARD

Dear Joshua,

I am writing to you to let you know how much of an impact you had on my father from the day he met you until his last few hours. Even when he forgot his family's names, he still referred to you by name. Even when we gave up, you kept pushing him. His quality of life was sustained through your help, guidance, and dedication.

Although my father was not a singer, he would always sing with you. Even though he had difficulty talking, he was able to sing a whole song. When you got him to speak again through song for my daughter on her wedding day, it was one of the most remarkable things I have ever seen.

You are a bright and inspiring person. I have never seen anyone light up a room of people with dementia the way you do. You told me you were going to change the industry, and I'm sure you will. Just keep doing what you do.

Juliette Simmons

This book is written primarily for caregivers of individuals with dementia. The information that is presented in this book can benefit anyone who wants to improve their understanding of dementia and the practical ways that we can improve the quality of life of those with dementia.

The Dementia Concept is structured in three parts. In Part 1, *Understand*, you will learn the signs, symptoms, and stages of dementia. This section provides an overview of the ways that those with dementia can maintain a vital connection to the world around them.

In Part 2, *Connect*, you will learn the core principles of connecting to individuals with dementia. Mindful interaction, conversation facilitation, creation of a routine, and the use of music as medicine can have profound impacts. Read examples of the successfulness of these methods.

In Part 3, *Engage*, you will learn to apply *The Dementia Concept* principles to even more specific events and interactions, and create a schedule to optimize each day. These holistic approaches to care have been repeatedly shown to benefit both individuals with dementia and the people who care for them.

Human nature drives us to continually seek new experiences throughout our lives. One of the most prevalent, false stigmas of dementia is that it signifies the end of learning. The reality is that people with dementia and other forms of memory impairment are capable of creating new memories and developing new skills. Although the type and severity of the dementia impacts these processes, there are ways to increase individual levels of success. The methods for interaction that are described in this book can be the difference between watching someone slip away and helping them remain engaged with their lives.

Caregivers and loved ones must recognize the importance of thoughtful and deliberate interaction. We must ask ourselves, "Who is this person? What do they love? How can we use our knowledge of what they love to help them engage with life?" It's not always easy to find a topic, object, or song that clicks with someone, but when you do, amazing things can happen. *The Dementia Concept* offers practical methods for engagement that serve to decrease agitation and increase success.

With consistency and repetition, we can help people with dementia to harness the power of Procedural Learning, which enables a new habit to be developed through the process of doing something over and over again. Procedural Learning is an important way for people with dementia to maintain and build upon their skills. In turn, they can increase their level of stability, productivity, independence, and happiness.

As caregivers, we often try to prevent people from making mistakes because we want to maximize their success. If we witness a person having trouble with something, we might decide it's best for us to do it for them. That approach effectively enables people in our care to lose their self-sufficiency. We might overlook the importance of daily self-care activities, commonly referred to as the Activities of Daily Living, such as getting ready for the day or making the bed, but these are essential elements of independence. We must allow time for people with dementia to attempt these tasks, even if they struggle. Doing so reinforces their skills and creates memories of new ways to approach challenges. If they struggle, we are there to provide support and guidance.

This book is based on a person-first approach to care. At its core is the understanding that people with dementia are still the same person they have always been, even though their needs and abilities are changing. Each person deserves a high level of respect and customized care. We must not reduce our perception of those for whom we care to the characteristics of dementia; we must continue to see them for who they are and tailor individualized care to suit their unique needs.

The Dementia Concept provides methods for engaging the whole individual, which results in a higher level of engagement. How can we use our knowledge of individual personalities to increase the quality of our connections? How can we make daily tasks and activities more enjoyable? *The Dementia Concept* describes approaches that make interactions more pleasant and successful by treating people with **understanding**, by **connecting** to what matters most to them, and by **engaging** them to be active participants in their own lives.

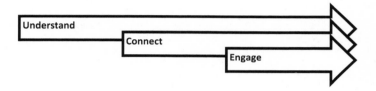

Part 1: Understand

The better we understand the form of dementia, its progression, and the available treatment options, the better quality of care we can provide.

CHAPTER ONE

Know the Facts

The term *dementia* refers to a classification of signs and symptoms. There are more than 100 types of dementia, of which Alzheimer's disease and Vascular dementia are the most commonly diagnosed types. Currently, over 5.5 million Americans are living with Alzheimer's disease, which constitutes 70 percent of the dementia population. This number is expected to triple within the next few decades.

Alzheimer's disease is one of the leading causes of death in the United States. One in three seniors die with Alzheimer's or another form of dementia.[1] Many researchers say that there is no cure in sight, and each year the number of cases grows worldwide. It is an epidemic that is soon to be classified as a pandemic. If a cure is not found within the next few decades, the rising cost of care could cripple the economy, and people living with dementia will

---

[1] Alzheimer's Association, 2014.

suffer from lack of funding for treatment options and caregiver education.

Fortunately, there is something that we can do to combat this problem through our work as caregivers. By increasing public awareness and improving caregiver education, we can help eliminate some of the detrimental stigmas associated with dementia. We must join the movement to change the way people with dementia and memory impairment are viewed and treated. *The Dementia Concept* offers a holistic, non-pharmacological approach to improving the quality of life of people with dementia. When this method is delivered with hopefulness and respect, it enables individuals to thrive. Increased understanding leads to better outreach and connection. In return, individuals with dementia can sustain and increase engagement with their lives.

CHAPTER TWO

Recognize the Myths

One of the myths associated with dementia is that it stops all new learning in its tracks. This myth overlooks the fact that Procedural Learning enables people with dementia to develop new memories. Human beings perceive and process information through two different avenues: propositional knowledge, which is the knowledge that we develop throughout our lives, and sensory-based knowledge, which is the information that we gain through our senses.

Dementia degenerates a person's propositional knowledge, and when that happens, the person becomes more reliant on sensory-based learning. Many people in the early stages of dementia rely heavily on propositional knowledge about their identity, preferences, values, and habits of behavior. As the dementia progresses, much of this unconscious knowledge is lost due to a decrease in neural activity. People are then faced with the challenge of an unfamiliar world. The subtext of their surroundings is diminished and must be reinterpreted at face value.

Imagine seeing an apple as a shiny, round, red object as opposed to interpreting many meanings from it, such as fruit is a healthy, edible food, and eating is necessary for our survival. Understanding that people with dementia may perceive their surroundings without some of its subtext can help us in our work as caregivers. We must provide them with the right amount of information and support to increase their success and reduce their confusion. (Part 2 of this book, *Connect,* will give you practical tools for tapping into sensory-based knowledge to support the needs of a person with dementia.)

Currently, society views people with dementia as people who can no longer do anything for themselves. This perception indicates that there is nothing that can be done to build upon the person's capabilities. This leads to a decrease in productivity and independence among people with dementia, as well as caregivers who think they must do everything for the person. Instead, people with dementia must be empowered to try. When we view the person as someone who can no longer do anything, the dementia progresses faster. Individuals learn to rely on the caregiver, which nurtures many of the characteristics of dementia and promotes more forgetfulness and physical inhibition. Remember this golden rule: allow the person to do as much as he or she can before you provide support. When assistance is needed, provide just enough to help that person be successful.

Stigmas about a person's abilities can be detrimental and damaging to that person's sense of self. In a series of one-on-one interviews that I conducted with a group of people with dementia, I posed a series of questions and recorded their feedback. The following response that I received from a woman named Josephine highlights this issue:

"I know I have a form of dementia. It has not stopped me from learning and exploring new things. The biggest struggle for me is the way the disease causes others to stereotype me. I am, and have always been, an independent woman. I get upset when some people try to shelter me from life. It makes me feel weak and dependent when my daughter tries to do everything for me."

The prevalent stereotypes that are associated with Alzheimer's and dementia are some of the primary reasons that people wait so long to speak with a doctor about their symptoms. Some people might think that a dementia diagnosis is the end of an active and fulfilling life, but it does not have to be. Remember Josephine's perspective when you are working with a person who has dementia. Strive to empower and support them to achieve as much as possible.

CHAPTER THREE

A Dementia Diagnosis is not the End

A diagnosis of dementia should not be viewed as the end of life. People can live with dementia for up to thirty years. We must empower people with dementia to continue to live purposefully. One major challenge is to educate the general public, healthcare providers, and medical personnel not to perpetuate the stigmas associated with dementia. We have the potential to improve quality of life through non-pharmacological, compensatory strategies for interaction. Although there is no cure for Alzheimer's disease or related dementias, in most cases there is a great deal that can be done to help people live active and fulfilling lives for a longer period of time.

The Dementia Concept offers techniques that treat the whole person, not just some of their symptoms. Through a combination of pharma-cological and non-pharmacological interventions, we can help people sustain awareness and promote neuroplasticity. Doing so naturally elevates mood, reinforces skills, and increases confidence. Neuroplasticity also reinforces the hippocampus, which is the part of the brain that directs memory, enabling people to create new memories and retain them longer.

The following graphic illustrates some aspects of our lives that are governed by the hippocampus and the amygdala, which is the part of the brain that governs sensory-based knowledge. We normally process information by using a combination of these evaluative processes. As dementia progresses, this scale tips so that more information is processed through sensory-based knowledge and the amygdala. Thus, gut feelings, a sense of purpose, and present experiences become more significant.

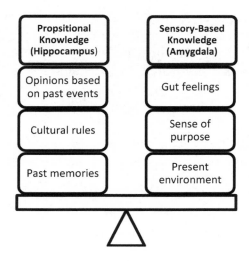

Many people who are diagnosed with dementia express fear of losing their independence. For many years, the dementia care community has overlooked the right of those with dementia to be active participants in their own care. More and more individuals are coming forward and demanding to have a say in what happens throughout the course of their dementia's progression.

When all medical decisions are made by a healthcare proxy and all financial decisions are made by the individual's Power of Attorney, this takes away the choice and the voice of individuals with dementia. To counteract this problem, the Alzheimer's Bill of Rights has been drafted to help people with dementia to foster a sense of independence. This Bill of Rights strongly reinforces their rights to be informed of their condition, given opportunities for engagement, and given a sense of independence within a safe, structured, and predictable environment.[2]

The care we provide must uphold these values. We must recognize the importance of engaging with the individual and making them a vital participant in their own healing.

---

[2] *The Best Friends Approach to Alzheimer's Care* by Virginia Bell and David Troxel. Copyright 1997, Health Professions Press, Inc.

CHAPTER FOUR

Signs and Symptoms

Different forms of dementia are classified by different signs and symptoms. Alzheimer's disease is very different from Vascular Dementia, which is very different from Frontotemporal Dementia, Lewy Body Dementia, and so on. Knowing which type of dementia a person has enables us to provide them with appropriate, personalized care. The better we understand the unique needs of any individual with whom we interact, the better friend we are to them, and the better we are able to provide high-quality support and interventions when necessary.

In this chapter, learn about some of the most common types of dementia, their characteristics, and helpful tips about what to expect and how to react. In recent years, the accuracy of diagnosis for different types of dementia has improved greatly. However, it is always important to get two professional opinions. Diagnosis is achieved through a combination of tests, including:

- Physical exam
- Neurological exam
- Complete Blood Count (CBC) test
- Blood chemistry screening
- Computed Tomography (CT) scan
- Positron Emission Tomography (PET) Scan
- Single-Photon Emission Computerized Tomography (SPECT) scan
- Functional Magnetic Resonance Imaging (fMRI)
- Magnetic Resonance Imaging (MRI)
- Sensory evaluation

If you or your loved one has been diagnosed with a form of dementia, have the results of these tests sent to an additional specialist to confirm the diagnosis. Doing so does not mean that you don't trust or respect your doctor; it means that you recognize the importance of a correct diagnosis, and you know that two minds are sometimes better than one.

The following is a summary of some of the most common types of dementia, the signs and symptoms by which they are classified, plus helpful hints for care. Keep in mind that every person is different and that symptoms may vary among individuals.

Alzheimer's disease (ALZ or AD) is the most common form of dementia. The first sign is typically mild memory loss, but, in many cases, the disease has been slowly progressing for years without any signs or symptoms. Over time, the brain atrophies and develops Amyloid Plaques and Neurofibrillary

Tangles, which degrade nerve cells and their interconnectivity.

Signs, Symptoms, and Characteristics:
- Short-term memory loss, progressing to long-term memory loss
- Repetition of questions and statements
- Inability to sequence events (confusion about what came first and what came last)
- Difficulty telling time on an analog clock
- Obsessive tendencies
- Difficulty communicating verbally
- Delayed physical responses
- Difficulty recognizing others
- Difficulty recognizing themselves in a mirror

Helpful Hints:
- Tap into long-term memories through the use of photos, stories, books, and music from the person's past.
- Use digital clocks instead of analog clocks.
- Increase engagement to reduce repetitive questions and statements. Boredom or lack of engagement can cause repetitive behavior.
- Keep the living environment clean and uncluttered.
- Harness obsessive tendencies by encouraging the person to help organize objects.
- If verbal communication is a challenge, try communicating through music. Singing

keeps our articulators in shape and sustains the physical ability to speak.
- When communicating, allow the person adequate time to process the information and respond.
- Reduce distraction and spatial confusion by limiting the number of mirrors in the living environment.

Vascular Dementia (VD), also known as Multi-Infarct Dementia (MID), is the second most common type of dementia. It is characterized by Transient Ischemic Attacks (TIAs), also known as mini-strokes, which cause inconsistent blood flow to the brain as well as fluctuating signs and symptoms.

Signs, Symptoms, and Characteristics:
- Inconsistent signs and symptoms that range from no symptoms to complete confusion
- Sleepwalking
- Paranoia
- Numb hands and feet

Helpful Hints:
- Over-exercising can increase confusion. Strive for light exercise once per day.
- Encourage the person to move their legs for a few minutes before standing up. If their legs are numb, they might have difficulty standing and walking.
- If the proper steps are taken, such as controlling blood pressure and regulating

blood sugar, skills and abilities may be sustained for a much longer period of time.

Frontotemporal Dementia (FTD) impairs one's ability to keep a routine and understand social cues. This makes it difficult, yet even more important, to maintain a structured schedule. When you change the daily routine of someone with FTD, the chances of that person exhibiting behavioral disturbances increases as does their confusion.

Signs, Symptoms, and Characteristics:
- Decreased attention span
- Saying whatever is on their mind
- Difficulty speaking in full sentences, often changing subjects mid-sentence
- Agitation with changes to, or lack of, daily schedule
- Rapidly progressing symptoms
- Behavioral changes that may mimic Bipolar Disorder or Schizophrenia

Helpful Hints:
- Use hand gestures alongside verbal communication.
- Use photos to help identify the person's surroundings, such as a photo of a toilet on the bathroom door and a photo of clothes on the closet door.
- Provide a nightlight in the bathroom and leave the bathroom door open.
- Place arrows on the inside of bedroom doors to provide directional cues:

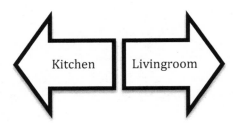

In the absence of cues like these, a person can become less inclined to venture out of their room. Remember that isolation can lead to apathy and depression. It is important to encourage people to engage with others and with their environment. Provide them with tools to make engagement easier to navigate.

Pick's Disease is a form of Frontotemporal Dementia. The signs and symptoms of Pick's Disease are the same as those of Frontotemporal Dementia, but Pick's Disease progresses at a much faster rate.

Lewy Body Dementia (LBD) is caused by a build-up of protein in the brain, known as Lewy bodies, which disrupt brain function. LBD is characterized by a lack of REM sleep, which can cause cognitive dysfunction, hallucination, and difficulty distinguishing dreams from reality.

Signs, Symptoms, and Characteristics:
- Hallucination
- Delusion

- Stiffness in the body, which may cause dragging of the feet, difficulty bending at the waist, and a shuffling gait
- Light to severe tremors
- Falls and fainting

Helpful Hints:
- Avoid negative news and other stimulus that can increase unpleasant hallucination and delusion.
- Provide thick-handled utensils and plate-guards to make eating easier.
- When walking with a person with LBD, stand on the side of their dominant hand to provide better support.
- Encourage them to lift their feet about 3 inches off the ground when walking to reinforce muscle memory.
- Marching music can be used to improve walking. Sing or play a marching song, such as "Off We Go into the Wild Blue Yonder" to help trigger rhythmic walking with lifted feet.
- When guiding someone to sit down, model the motion for them, encouraging them to bend at the hip.

Creutzfeldt-Jakob disease (CJD) is a rare brain disorder in which dementia progresses rapidly. It causes memory failure, behavioral changes, lack of coordination, and visual disturbances. Mental deterioration, involuntary movements, weakness of extremities, blindness, and coma might occur in the later stages.

Signs, Symptoms, and Characteristics:
- Frequent fluctuation in the ability to recall memories
- Stubbornness, argumentativeness, tendency to attempt emotional manipulation
- Delusion, hallucination, and paranoia

Helpful Hints:
- People with CJD are often motivated to help others, so invite them to read to someone or help set the table.
- Spirituality often appeals to people with CJD. Attending services or providing inspirational reading material can be soothing and engaging for some people.
- Respond to argumentativeness or emotional manipulation with reassurance and validation. Tell the person that you understand, and you're there to help.

CHAPTER FIVE

Symptom Progression

Did you know that as we age, we lose our abilities in the order opposite that which they are gained in childhood? This is exhibited most notably by people with dementia. A newborn baby will grasp your finger when it is in front of them, and this is an ability that is often retained even at the hour of our death. The first five skills we learn usually remain with us into the final stages of our lives.

Graphic on next page

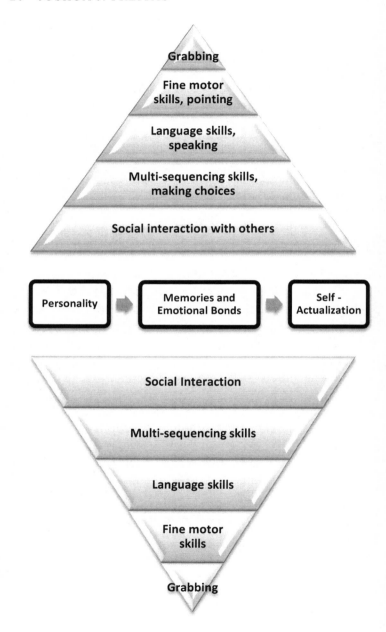

It's important to know and respect people's capabilities. Not doing so can cause harm. Now that you have a better understanding of the signs, symptoms, and characteristics of the most common types of dementia, learning about the progression of dementia will help you identify someone's ability throughout each stage.

Let's consider symptom progression with an example of someone who loves to cook. In the early stages, the person might be able to cook almost entirely on their own. As they progress into mid-stages, they might be able to help by stirring or serving food if they are assisted with cues and support. A person in a later stage would need almost total assistance, but they may still enjoy the texture and the smell of something like cookie dough in their hands. Remember that people in later stages of dementia rely heavily on sensory-based knowledge and experiences, much as we do when we are very young. Although someone's role in activities may change, they can still enjoy aspects of the activity and the interactive experience.

Everyone is different, and people may experience different symptoms that progress at different rates. However, the industry standard is to identify the progression of dementia through 7 distinct stages that are based on a system developed by Barry Reisberg, M.D., clinical director of the NYU School of Medicine's Silberstein Aging and Dementia Research Center.

Dementia Stage 1

In this stage, information processing is primarily normal, and information is accessed from both propositional and sensory-based knowledge. Symptoms of this stage might be subtle enough that medical professionals do not see the signs or symptoms. A person in this stage may experience occasional confusion; increased anxiety; altered speech; mood swings; personality changes; wandering; changes in blood pressure and heart rate; mild delusions, and inaccurate recollection of the immediate past.

Dementia Stage 2

In this stage, a person will experience a noticeable cognitive impairment. This decline may seem to be part of the normal aging process, but its onset is sudden. Normal brain function and information processing continues through both propositional and sensory-based knowledge. A person in this stage of dementia may experience memory lapses; mild aphasia (difficulty recalling words); frequently losing or misplacing objects; slight social withdrawal.

Dementia Stage 3

In this stage, cognitive decline, although still mild, may become noticeable by friends, family, and coworkers. Medical professionals may be able to identify problems with memory or concentration through cognitive testing. Information processing may begin to shift to sensory-based knowledge as a primary method with the secondary support of propositional knowledge. A person in this stage of dementia may experience mild to moderate aphasia and difficulty remembering new people's names; difficulty performing tasks in social and work settings; difficulty with reading comprehension; losing or misplacing valuable objects; difficulty with planning, organization, and sequencing.

Dementia Stage 4

In this stage, a person may experience moderate cognitive decline, which medical professionals can diagnose by observing specific symptoms in several areas. Information is processed primarily through the senses with the limited support of propositional knowledge. A person in this stage of dementia may experience short-term memory loss; long-term memory loss; inability to do basic math; inability to manage medication; moodiness and social withdrawal, especially in socially or cognitively challenging situations; changes in personality exhibited by new and uncharacteristic behaviors, such as singing or dancing in public.

Dementia Stage 5

In this stage, moderate to severe cognitive decline occurs alongside extremely noticeable forgetfulness. A person in this stage may begin to need help with the activities of daily living, such as putting toothpaste on a toothbrush or folding clothes, but they can still perform some tasks independently, such as feeding themselves and using the bathroom. Information is processed primarily through sensory-based learning with almost no propositional knowledge.

A person in this stage may experience inability to recall their address, telephone number, middle name, hometown, or other details about themselves; increased confusion about where they are or where they have been recently; inability to tell time; need for assistance with daily planning such as choosing food, clothing, and activities; difficulty navigating their living environment, remembering where different rooms are, and where objects belong.

Dementia Stage 6

In this stage, a person may experience severe and progressive cognitive decline. Information is processed primarily through sensory-based experiences with little or no propositional knowledge. The person may need hand-under-hand assistance[3] with the activities of daily living and may experience an inconsistent ability to perform tasks. A person in this stage may experience major changes in sleep patterns; severe difficulty with motor-skill based tasks and dressing without supervision, commonly exhibiting self-securing behavior by putting on multiple layers of clothing. A person in this stage likely requires assistance with self-care such as meal planning, eating, bathing, and using the bathroom.

---

[3] The hand-under-hand assistance method is described in Chapter 11, Approaches to Interaction.

Dementia Stage 7

A person in the final stage of dementia experiences progressive and severe cognitive decline. Information is processed through sensory-based experiences with no propositional knowledge. A person in this stage loses the ability to respond to their environment and verbally participate in conversation. They will eventually lose fine motor skills, such as the ability to grasp, as well as mobility, including the ability to twist or turn (gross-trunk movement). A wheelchair is required. A person in this stage may experience the need for assistance to accomplish everyday tasks; inability to communicate verbally; difficulty eating, necessitating a soft or liquid diet; and increased need or desire for sleep.

Remember that quality of life can always be improved for people with dementia, even in the advanced stages. Although they may lose the ability to communicate verbally, they may like to be talked to. Although they may lose independent mobility, they may enjoy being taken for a walk in their wheelchair. They may no longer be capable of planning and coordinating their daily tasks and transitions, but they will benefit from a caregiver who offers compassionate support in these areas.

Use cues to lessen agitation when you are guiding someone through tasks and transitions. Radiate an encouraging attitude. Consider the power of the words you choose, the tone you use, and the ability for music to soothe. These techniques will strengthen your ability to be the kind of caregiver and friend who can help others find happiness, even when they are struggling.

CHAPTER SIX

Holistic Treatments

Most forms of dementia do not currently have a cure, but they all have treatment options, including both pharmacological and non-pharmacological approaches and interventions. Unfortunately, there are misconceptions associated with pharmacological treatment. Many people believe medication that is used to treat dementia symptoms slows down dementia's progression. In reality, medications are only a temporary mask for the signs and symptoms,[4] just as an antihistamine can clear up congestion but cannot cure the flu.

Often, families keep their loved one on medication after it has stopped working because they hope that the medication has curative power. This is a costly and potentially dangerous misconception. Over-medicating can cause a secondary form of medically-induced dementia

---

[4] Alzheimer's Association, 2014.
http://www.alz.org/research/science/alzheimers_disease_treatments.asp

known as delirium. Delirium is marked by increased confusion, depression, agitation, and it may speed the progression of the initially diagnosed condition. Delirium is often caused by the Medicine Cascade Effect (MCE) which is when one medication is prescribed to treat another medication's side effect. MCE can compromise cerebral capacity and, thus, the individual's ability to think. If MCE is not identified promptly, it may cause permanent damage. In addition to MCE, over-medication can cause fatigue, increased memory impairment, difficulty reasoning, impaired balance, increased chance of falling, and the potential for bad drug interactions.

Reliance on medication for the treatment of dementia has risks, such as receiving the wrong medication due to a misdiagnosis of the type of dementia. Since Alzheimer's disease is the most common form of dementia, it is often the fallback diagnosis when the actual type of dementia is unclear. That is a dangerous fact because if, for example, a person with Lewy Body dementia is misdiagnosed as having Alzheimer's disease, improper medication can cause severe side effects including worsening symptoms, sedation, tremors, and permanent damage to the brain that can even be fatal.

Pharmacological interventions can have positive outcomes, such as helping someone with social anxiety, clinical depression, and difficulty focusing. But these benefits do not always outweigh the medical risks or the social and financial expense of pharmacological reliance. The best approach to treating dementia is to combine medication that works with holistic, non-pharmacological care.

Non-pharmacological interventions for dementia, such as expressive arts therapy, music therapy, social engagement, and exercise, have the ability to treat the whole person. These are holistic treatments because they treat the whole person and take mental and social factors into account instead of only the physical symptoms. These holistic treatments have been proven to cause significant improvements to overall well-being and sustained cognitive function. Holistic treatment approaches can increase neuroplasticity, physical functionality, fine motor skills, and even eyesight. In many cases, if a person is engaged in social, physical, emotional, and intellectual activity, dementia's progression slows.

Despite a tremendous amount of research supporting the effectiveness of non-pharmacological treatments, there are many healthcare providers that do not recognize the validity of these approaches. In many cases, their resistance is due to the false belief that people with dementia can't get better. One might ask, "If there is no hope for a complete cure, then why bother?" We must not think this way, because there is hope for improvement. Life is made up of a series of moments, and each moment matters. If we have the ability to improve just one day in someone else's life by connecting with them authentically, then we should. The beauty of this approach is that, when used consistently, multi-disciplinary holistic methods have the transformative power to improve an individual's condition, as in the following example.

Mr. Smith was in the mid-stages of Vascular dementia. He had lived in a nursing home for two years and had exhibited extreme agitation and combative behaviors like hitting and spitting, which caused Mr. Smith to be put on medication. After spending time with him and finding out that he enjoyed fishing, we presented Mr. Smith with a tackle-box and hook-removed fishing gear. After a few minutes, Mr. Smith started to talk about fishing, and he did not exhibit any concerning behaviors. We had found something that helped him connect and engage in a way that was meaningful to him.

Observing the interest Mr. Smith showed in the tackle-box made us realize that it could be used as an effective therapy tool. Whenever Mr. Smith was lonely, sad, or agitated, we provided him with the tackle-box to redirect his attention. We added some interactive tools to the box, including conversation questions such as, "Where is your favorite place to go fishing?" and "What kind of bait would you use to catch a large fish?"[5] We also used the tackle-box to engage Mr. Smith in a sorting game of organizing, matching, and describing each object in the box. The tackle-box became an inspiration for supervised fishing outings. Although we didn't supply Mr. Smith with fishing hooks, he enjoyed casting out the line of his own fishing rod. Within weeks, procedural learning enabled Mr. Smith to use the tackle-box on

---

[5] This is a form of Conversation Quilting, a *Dementia Concept* method that is further described in Chapter 14.

his own whenever he chose to, and it became part of his daily routine. The tackle-box tool improved

Mr. Smith's skills with emotional coping, communication, and independence.

Soon after beginning this form of therapy with an object of interest, Mr. Smith moved from a residential care facility into an assisted living community, and after a week of living there, he had not exhibited any concerning behaviors. Throughout the month that followed, I was involved in planning Mr. Smith's ongoing care. He continued to improve and did not exhibit the combative behaviors that had caused him to be medicated, so he was able to stop taking that medication. These behavioral improvements were achieved by the non-pharmacological approach to care that appealed to and inspired him as an individual. This approach seems simple, but it is often profoundly effective.

Although medication has its place, we need to think outside the box. Medication that is prescribed for one symptom of dementia is often combined with other medications to deal with other symptoms, which can result in dangerous drug interactions and over-medication. Holistic, non-pharmacological interventions, on the other hand, can be completely safe, cost effective, and have a tremendous number of benefits that should be embraced rather than overlooked.

CHAPTER SEVEN

Activating Neuroplasticity

Neuroplasticity is a term that refers to changes in the brain, throughout our lives, as a result of our behavior. Our environment, thoughts, emotions, and relationships influence the firing of our synapses along neural pathways in the brain. When the brain has suffered an injury or is affected by dementia, therapeutic approaches can be used to help the brain reroute the synaptic network of information-processing. This enables the brain to compensate for areas that are not working. Plasticity is the brain's ability to detour around an injured part of the brain to find new ways to perform lost skills.

With every challenge comes an opportunity. A dementia diagnosis is no exception. In a supportive environment with the right approaches to care, people with dementia can improve neuroplasticity. Doing so can improve their cognitive abilities and slow the progression of their condition.

Parts of the brain grow and strengthen like a muscle when they are used and challenged continuously. Knowing that people with dementia can still learn through sensory-based experiences and Procedural Learning, we must continue to allow them to experience life to whatever degree they're most able. Finding ways to overcome challenges has a positive effect on the brain. When individuals are encouraged, supported, and empowered to find the strength within themselves to overcome challenges, the result is a stronger brain.

Take, for example, London's fleet of taxi drivers, who do not use GPS or any other navigational devices. They rely on training and memory, which is developed through Procedural Learning. They drive different routes across the streets of London over and over again until they have committed the map to memory. During this process, the taxi driver's hippocampus actually grows in size as a result of continuous learning. The same result is possible for people with dementia. If they are in an environment where they are encouraged and enabled to continue learning, they can strengthen and build upon their existing cognitive function.

CHAPTER EIGHT

Different Types of Learning

There are many different types of learning that can be used in simple ways to promote neuroplasticity. Actively engage in activities that trigger the following types of learning: physical, experiential, novelty, and emotional.

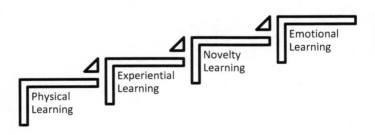

Physical Learning through exercise and behavioral tasks can increase blood-flow and foster more neural activity. Repetition of a physical action also reinforces muscle memory, making these tasks easier to perform over time.

Examples:
- Going for a walk
- Morning or evening stretching
- Completing a daily self-care routine, such as tooth-brushing and face-washing
- Organizing objects in the living environment

Experiential Learning fosters focused attention, which physically changes the brain, increases social participation, and generates multi-sensory stimulation.

Examples:
- Going to a museum
- Shopping for groceries
- Aerobic exercise
- Cooking or watching someone cook, smelling the food, and feeling the textures

Novelty learning, or learning new things, creates new neural pathways throughout the brain, which can bypass injured areas.

Examples:
- Going on vacation
- People-watching
- Learning words in a new language
- Staying engaged with popular culture

Emotional Learning is the process of learning things that get filtered through the amygdala, the part of the brain that processes sensory experiences and emotions. This often occurs during major life events that have emotional significance.

Examples:
- Going to a wedding
- Attending a concert or musical
- Meeting a new baby
- Attending a spiritual or religious service
- Doing something that invokes laughter

**When one skill is lost,
another skill is strengthened.**

Throughout the progression of dementia, there is a noticeable change in the *nature of knowing*, the way an individual processes and perceives information about the world around them. The brain has a miraculous ability to adapt to changes and compensate for lost skills. Instead of focusing on the skills that are lost, encourage those who are affected by dementia to recognize all that they're able to do. Bringing attention to our abilities, rather than our inabilities, promotes and nurtures positive outcomes.

To help a person sustain their skills, we must focus on what they can do, then continually reinforce those skills. Look for the areas of competence and engagement that are still intact. Strive to engage the individual in those areas and build upon them. A person may no longer be as skilled at conversation or as physically agile as they once were, but they are still processing the world around them in other ways, such as through art, music, and their emotions.

In some parts of the world, dementia treatment consists of medicating a person and locking them away. In other parts of the world, elderly individuals are embraced as valued members of society. In those places, dementia treatment is driven by the goal to provide care that keeps the person engaged with society for as long as possible. This should be the worldwide goal. We must increase and share the knowledge that life with dementia is still valuable and can be filled with learning and connection. Understanding this can break the stigmas that too often obstruct quality care.

When one skill is lost, a compensatory skill is often gained. Harvard University Professor Howard Gardner's theory of Multiple Intelligences[6] reminds us that everyone has different natural aptitudes: visual, interpersonal, intrapersonal, linguistic, logical-mathematical, musical, spatial, and physical. As our strengths lessen in some areas, we can cultivate aptitudes in other areas. This is a more optimistic outlook than checking off the skills that have been lost; and remember, optimism invites success. Tasks that require logical-mathematical intelligence may be challenging due to the loss of propositional knowledge; however, sensory-based intelligence may increase. Musical intelligence often increases to compensate for the loss of logical-mathematical or linguistic aptitude. Use this knowledge to connect and engage through different types of activities that appeal to multiple types of intelligence.

---

[6] Howard Gardner, www.multipleintelligencesoasis.org

Part 2: Connect

When the quality of our connection with others improves, so does our quality of life.

CHAPTER NINE

Staying Connected

We often forget that communication is not only verbal. For someone with dementia, good communication can be a simple touch or receiving a thoughtful compliment to break the ice. During interactions, remember that connection and engagement are the goals. Connection with others is essential to an optimal quality of life, especially for those with dementia, who face a high risk of isolation and depression.

You might find that some people with dementia often decline to participate in activities, and we must respect their preferences. If someone does not feel like participating then they have the right to decline. Regardless of how many times a person declines participation, we should always invite them with the hope that on some days they will decide to participate.

There are ways to engage even the most withdrawn people, increase their participation, and help them to communicate more effectively. The following chapters offer techniques for how to connect effectively in order to bring out the best in others.

CHAPTER TEN

The Four Dimensions of Sustainability

The Four Dimensions of Sustainability is a model for connecting with the whole person by interacting through physical, social, cognitive, and emotional experiences. Connecting with people who are living with dementia across these four dimensions has been proven to generate many positive outcomes, including increased overall engagement with life, reduced confusion, and reduced agitation. A person with dementia may be unable to fully recover, but a multifaceted approach to interaction can help slow or even reverse the progression of some signs and symptoms.

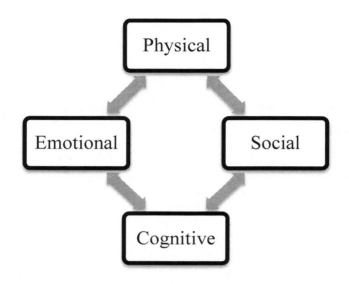

Physical Sustainability

Exercise can have a positive ripple effect throughout the day and is linked to improved mood in both patients and caregivers. Exercise releases endorphins, which reduce pain and increase feelings of happiness. Exercise increases dexterity and reduces the pain associated with arthritis, which affects 50 percent of people over the age of 65. Exercise can reinforce muscle memory, improve sociability, and reduce agitation and depression. 50 percent of people living with dementia also suffer from depression, so it is important to avoid the factors that increase the odds, such as social withdrawal and physical inactivity.

Research also shows that regular exercise can help prevent dementia, improve cognitive functionality, and support the development of new neural pathways. Remaining physically active improves observable aspects of brain function, including concentration, the ability to create and maintain new memories, and increased stability of mood and behavior.

Social Sustainability

To maintain meaning in our lives, we must continuously engage with others and explore our world. Our human spirit of interpersonal and self-exploration is what makes us different from other animals. We are curious about how and why things work, how aspects of our lives make us feel, and how to communicate our feelings to others. Keeping these values in mind makes it easier to engage someone with dementia in a meaningful way that keeps them wanting to learn and connect.

Social interaction decreases the signs and symptoms of dementia and the challenging behaviors that are caused by lack of understanding. Maintaining social relationships and engagement with peers can validate one's feelings and reduce isolation, stress, apathy, and depression.

For many people, spiritual engagement is an important form of social engagement. It can be one way to recognize that our lives have meaning and purpose. Understanding that our lives are an ever-evolving journey can bring peace to those who are struggling to cope with dementia. Connecting to spirituality can also bring people with common interests together in a supportive way that inspires inner peace. These benefits can decrease apathy, isolation, frustration, and depression.

We all need to feel a sense of purpose. What would the world be like without it? For the vast majority of people, our sense of purpose is related to our sense of ourselves in relation to others. What roles do we play? Where, and with whom, do we belong? Creating a sense of purpose for someone with dementia instills a sense of belonging. It identifies and proclaims a need for that person in the world. For someone with dementia, being able to play a role, complete a task, help others, and receive thanks gives them the opportunity to be important and independent. Helping is a behavior that releases serotonin both in caregivers and the people for whom they care. Finding ways for people with dementia to collaborate in service to others can be a worthwhile endeavor for everyone.

Cognitive Sustainability

We are all born with an intense desire to learn more about aspects of the world that interest us. This sense of curiosity and the ability to learn is still present among those with dementia. It is important to engage that curiosity. When people continuously learn new things, they improve cognitive function by increasing neuroplasticity and reinforcing the hippocampus. Memories can be strengthened and skills can be sustained.

Since people with dementia can continue to learn through Procedural Learning, cognitive engagement is an important way to get a person with dementia to take part in the ever-changing world around them. Intellectual engagement also fosters relationships that are based on personal interests among both patients and caregivers, which creates a stronger interpersonal connection and a better continuum of care.

Emotional Sustainability

As we gain a better understanding of how people who are living with dementia process information, we observe their enduring ability to process emotions. Dementia often takes away the ability to communicate verbally, but through activities such as art-based expression, people with dementia can process emotional challenges in a healthy way.

During and after art-based expression, people with dementia are more at ease and better able to cope due an increase of dopamine. Dopamine is a natural chemical that helps control the brain's reward and pleasure centers, which help people relax. Isn't it amazing that our bodies have the ability to produce these powerful remedies without the use of pharmaceuticals? Sometimes all it takes to overcome a challenging moment is some artistic creativity. Connecting with others through creative and artistic activities is just one form of emotional engagement that increases communication and reduces depression.

The following chapters offer practical, hands-on approaches for implementing these principles.

CHAPTER ELEVEN

Approaches to Interaction

The way we approach people, guide them, listen, and respond to them influences the success of our conversations and interactions. Make compassion your primary intention, and use the following practical approaches to interaction when caring for someone with dementia.

Here are seven steps for mindful connection that help to create transitions, routine, and a sense of purpose.

1. **Introduce yourself to the person, and provide prompting information.**

   "Hi, I'm Joshua, and I will be your caregiver today." Or, *"Hi, Mom; it's your son, Josh. I'm here to visit you."*

2. **When communicating, make eye contact and communicate at the person's eye-level.**

3. **Give a compliment, and then invite the person to help or participate.**

   "I bet you're great at this activity. Would you like to join us?" Or, *"I could really use your help with this; will you help me?"*

4. **When offering choices, provide no more than two or three options.**

   "Would you like to join us for morning exercise, or would you rather read the newspaper?"

5. **Provide the person with something to hold for comfort.**

   The sensory experience of holding something releases dopamine, increase a sense of calm and comfort. Holding an object can also improve engagement and focus.

   During activities, try offering a small pillow or another favorite object.

6. **Sit groups in a circle or side-by-side.**

   Everyone should be a front-row learner. If you sit side-by-side with someone with dementia, sit on the side of their dominant hand.

7. **Provide a clear ending to activities by thanking the participants and creating an emotional and physical connection.**

"Thank you for singing with me today!" Offer each person a handshake or a hug.

The following approaches offer more methods for achieving successful interaction. They prioritize kindness, compassion, and patience, which are qualities that can improve your relationship with anyone.

Give More Compliments

Compliment Therapy is the act of pointing out the positive attributes that you see in someone. When someone receives a sincere compliment, it reinforces positive self-esteem and increases positive behaviors. Compliments can cause endorphins to be released in the recipient's brain. You will see a brightening of the expression, a lightening of the spirit, and an increase in energy. Even after a specific compliment is forgotten, an emotional bond endures.

When you initiate interaction by giving a compliment, you instill a sense of confidence, belonging, and trust. Start conversations with statements like, "Mrs. Smith, what's your secret to staying so beautiful?" or "Joe, you have a handshake like a president!" Human beings are more likely to agree and comply with those who compliment us, even if that compliment is as simple as someone remembering our name. Giving compliments makes it easier to manage difficult behaviors that might arise during an interaction.

Listen compassionately and validate feelings

We all have a desire for our feelings to be validated by others. When connecting with someone with dementia, it is important to validate how he or she is feeling.

Start conversations by acknowledging the person's countenance, for example, *"Hi, Mom; it's me, Josh! You seem happy today."* Or, if someone seems markedly upset, validate that by saying, *"Hi, Mr. Smith; you seem sad. Would you like to talk to me?"* Let the person know that you are there to help.

Validating another person's feelings is a way of establishing a meaningful connection with them. Show the person that you care and are willing to listen. Use this connection to direct the conversation toward assessing what support they need and attempting to provide it.

Match emotion to emotion

If someone is feeling sad, you should match your emotion with theirs. Put yourself in their shoes. If you were visibly upset and a friend approached you with smiles and laughter without asking you what was wrong, might you feel disregarded and invisible? The same is true for someone with dementia, and sometimes even more so, because verbal and cognitive obstacles can make it more challenging for them to express their feelings. We must match and mirror their emotional state: sad with sad and happy with happy. Connecting with their emotional experience is a form of empathy that gives you a chance to help redirect the emotion.

If Mr. Smith seems sad and lonely, walk over to him and validate his feelings. Ask if you can sit with him for a few minutes. Mirror his emotional demeanor when you speak to him. This will comfort him and enable you to begin asking more questions about how he feels and what might make him feel better. Throughout the conversation, you will notice that Mr. Smith will also start to mirror your emotional demeanor. Use this opportunity to lighten his mood and slowly bring the conversation to a happier place. Redirect the topic to something other than loneliness, and see if you can engage him in a connected social activity.

Appeal to All Five Senses

As dementia progresses, sensory-based learning begins to take a primary role in cognitive processing. Instead of focusing on a person's loss of propositional knowledge, we can leverage their ability to stay connected to the world through their senses.

Taste: Provide little tastes of food before dinner to communicate to the brain that dinner is approaching.

Smell: Appetizing smells in the kitchen signify that the kitchen is a place for food. Encourage people to smell food before eating it. Encourage them to take deep breaths in the garden when you take them for a walk. Smell is highly linked to memory and keeping the nose engaged can help maintain connections to stored memories.

Touch: Sensory-based knowledge gives us a gateway for connection through touch. Encourage people to feel the objects they are working with, and provide them access to objects that they can manipulate.

Hearing: We must often speak louder to be heard by older people, but remember to use a loud, clear talking voice rather than a yelling voice. A gentle, mellow tone can be calming, and a hostile or impatient tone can be threatening and agitating.

Sight: Use color deliberately to create a more welcoming, stimulating, or calming environment.[7] Use lighting to convey cues about the time of day.

The 15-minute rule

Have patience. It takes a person with dementia about 15 minutes to become acclimated to his or her surroundings, after which the windows of opportunity for meaningful interaction will begin to widen. The average brain tends to process information differently about every 15 minutes, and

---

[7] The use of color is further described in Chapter 18, Engaging Through Color.

interestingly, the average attention span of a person with dementia is typically about 15 minutes. Remember to give people 15 minutes to acclimate to new surroundings and another 15 minutes to begin to participate. Your patience during transitions will truly help them engage with the next activity.

If a person with dementia starts to exhibit a concerning behavior, give him or her about 15 minutes before attempting to redirect the behavior. This allows the brain to process the information you are giving them with a different set of neurotransmitters.

Hand-under-hand

When you must guide someone physically, the approach matters. The *hand-under-hand* approach for physical assistance uses your hand to perform a task while the person you're guiding rests their hand on top of yours. This enables the person you're guiding to feel what your hands are doing, so that they can perform the action with your support. This is a non-invasive method to hands-on helping that assists rather than forces.

The *hand-under-hand* approach can be used as a meaningful method to social connection while also giving assistance during tasks such as dining and the many other activities of daily living. The use of this method can be particularly effective during bathing to reduce anxiety and resistance.

Hand-over-hand

The *hand-over-hand* approach helps a person complete a task with forced direction. The caregiver guides a person's hand to complete an action with limited help from the person. This is an invasive approach that forces rather than assists. Remember to handle people gently and offer them lots of supportive reassurance. When used correctly, this technique can lead to a positive emotional result. It can create a memory of having completed an action that has become impossible. This technique uses the healing power of touch to bypass the parts of the brain that have been damaged by dementia.

CHAPTER TWELVE

Connecting to our Living Environment

In the Netherlands, there is a living community called The Dementia Village.[8] It is home to over 150 people who are living with memory impairment. They live in lifestyle groups that are formed around their mutual interests. The architecture and decor of the living spaces are carefully designed to suit the needs of each individual lifestyle and to make the purpose of each space as clear as possible to those by whom it is occupied.

The Dementia Village is a gated community that has coffee shops, grocery stores, activity halls, and more. Every employee is trained to work with dementia, from the taxi drivers to the grocery store employees. Money is never exchanged; payment is billed to the resident's account. Each resident in the community has their own home with a bedroom,

---

[8] Dementia Village, www.dementiavillage.com.

bathroom, and kitchen free of potentially dangerous appliances.

As a result of their environment, residents of The Dementia Village decline up to five times more slowly, without medication, compared to the average. The environment enables, encourages, and stimulates independence and continued engagement with life. The Dementia Village exemplifies the concept of a supportive, non-pharmacological approach to dementia care, and it has had tremendous measurable outcomes.

"One of the things that creates comfort for people who have trouble thinking is space," my dear friend Alan Hochberg told me. "If you are too blocked in, you feel frightened." A person's living environment, whether it is an assisted living facility, nursing home, or private home, should reinforce a sense of openness, purpose, family, and community. There are benefits to living environments with simple layouts and simple design. Cluttered spaces can cause confusion and create physical obstacles.

One's living environment serves as a secure platform from which other experiences can spring forth. An environment of normality is a term we use to describe a consistent and nurturing living environment. Only after starting with the baseline of a stable and normalized living environment can individuals excel in their daily lives. Most of us take for granted our ability to cope with the amount of change and physical stimulation that we experience every day. For someone who is struggling to make sense of the world, an environment that is not in sync with their lifestyle can be disruptive. When the living environment is appropriately designed, and a behavioral routine is established, an individual's ability to confidently explore new things increases. And as we've discussed, learning new things keeps us feeling connected and engaged with our lives.

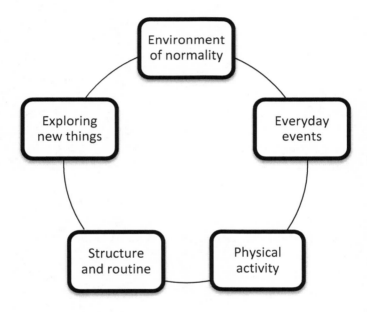

Provide a welcoming environment where people can continue to learn, explore, and sustain life skills. This will improve their quality of life through making the activities of daily living easier to complete. Continuously provide opportunities for engagement through a vast selection of person-centric, therapeutic, and research-based opportunities that we will continue to discuss and guide you through in this book.

Keep objects that the individual needs to access within their view. A toothbrush in a toothbrush-holder next to the bathroom sink is much more easily found than one that is kept inside a medicine cabinet. Prevent the agitation and frustration that can occur when essential objects are hidden or inaccessible.

Keep in mind that the living environment should feel neither restricted nor unsafe. It should be tailored to the level of support that the individual requires. An effort should be made to normalize any changes to the environment that are required due to an increased need for care. Instead of locking drawers and doors to prevent access to hazards, put those materials somewhere that is out of sight or reach. Locks on cabinets, drawers, and doors can make someone with dementia feel locked in or restricted, which may result in challenging behaviors or exit-seeking.

When thinking about the person's living environment, remember the goal: to reinforce a sense of comfort, stability, and calm. Imagine the unease that you might feel if you attempted to open a cabinet in your home but found it to be unexpectedly locked. Allow freedom for exploration in a way that ensures safety. Think about the small changes that you can make to reduce danger without imposing restrictions, such as replacing a multipurpose cleaning product with a spray-bottle full of vinegar. Vinegar can clean just as well, but it is non-toxic. Small changes such as this can have big impacts on safety and behavior.

Safety is something we all strive for: we wear seatbelts in a car, we wear bicycle helmets when riding a bike, and we wear sunscreen when we are out in the sun. There will always be risks associated with life no matter how hard we try to avoid them, so the best we can do is take the proper precautions. Be aware of the risks relevant to people with dementia, and put safety measures in place to help avoid accidents. Safety is what we strive for, but our ability to cope with life's risks and proceed in spite of them is what courage is all about.

Environment

A room with small area rugs, clutter, or too much furniture increases the likelihood of slips, trips, and falls. Some simple solutions can include organizing and removing clutter, rearranging or removing furniture, applying adhesives to keep area rugs and carpeting in place, or removing small area rugs altogether. When implementing these simple solutions try not to go overboard: a big change in environment can trigger confusion. Again, the goal is always for the environment to be as welcoming, comforting, and safe as possible.

Perception

Visual impairment affects three out of four people over the age of 65. When you add visual impairment, the level of risk can be very high. Objects such as rubber bands, marbles, flowers, or game pieces can be mistaken for candy or snacks. Proactive solutions to lower the risks include eliminating these objects altogether, keeping them to a minimum, or replacing them with low-risk objects. Replace a toxic flower or plant with a non-toxic one, or keep objects such as marbles and rubber bands somewhere safe where they can be used with extra support and guidance.

Lighting

Increasing the amount of lighting in the person's living environment can improve visibility and decrease the chance of a fall. Nightlights in the hallways, bedrooms, and bathrooms illuminate the way when it is dark. Lighting can also be used to increase awareness about the time of day. Make sure people have plenty of access to natural light during the day, and be mindful of the amount of artificial light that they are exposed to in the evening. An excessive amount of light before bedtime can disrupt the circadian rhythm which affects our quality of sleep.

Household Hazards

Basic appliances and household objects can become dangerous. Take precautions to help ensure that these items do not put people at risk. Make sure small appliances in the living environment, such as coffee makers or toaster ovens, are equipped with automatic shut-off features. Put sharp knives or cooking utensils out of sight and reach.

If supplements and prescription medications are to be administered under supervision, remove them from the kitchen table, counters, and medicine cabinet. Medications and dangerous chemicals, such as bleach or other caustic cleansers, should be kept out of sight and reach at all times. Dangerous chemicals can be replaced with non-toxic or all-natural options.

Organization

Put things where people would expect them to be such as cookies in a cookie jar, rather than loose change; coats in the coat closet, not on a chair in the bedroom. Use labels and signs to help keep things organized and identifiable. Put items that the person needs to access in the open where they can be seen.

CHAPTER THIRTEEN

Remind-Routine-Reward

Exercising the brain by learning and exploring new things promotes neuroplasticity and improves the likelihood of storing new memories. When you are responsible for coordinating the lifestyle of someone with dementia, be sure to offer engaging and varied activities. New and engaging activities enable a person with dementia to stay connected to other people and the world around them.

Many people believe that brain games keep the brain sharp, but recent research shows that this is not entirely accurate. The best brain games are those that include a component of consistently performing new tasks, whereas repetitive brain games may only improve success at completing one particular task. Learning and doing new things enables the brain to develop new neural pathways.

New skills and information have many benefits, but the best benefit is derived from combining new skills with the creation of new routines. Consistently challenging the brain to master a new skill is associated with the highest rate of brain stimulation. There are lots of real-life ways to continually challenge the brain. Things such as writing with your non-dominant hand, learning how to play an instrument, or learning phrases in another language are good examples of activities that promote neuroplasticity.

For a person with dementia, remember that a new skill or habit may take longer to develop, but it can be achieved with the remind-routine-reward cycle. Provide reminders to help people with dementia form new routines, and reinforce their participation in new activities with praise and rewarding encouragement. In time, the remind-routine-reward cycle can motivate an individual to move outside of their comfort zone to overcome challenges. Doing so improves that individual's level of successful independence.

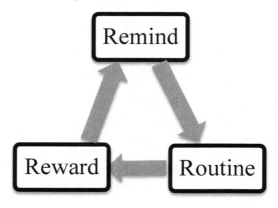

Consider the simple example of reminding someone to brush their teeth for 35 consecutive days. 35 days is the average length of time that it takes for a person with dementia to create a new habit or routine. The reward is cleaner teeth and a sense of independence. Continued reminders and regular brushing equates a new, healthy habit.

CHAPTER FOURTEEN

Quilting a Conversation

Quilting a conversation is a *Dementia Concept* technique for facilitating better communication between those with dementia, their caregivers, and their peers. Quilting a conversation joins at least two social topics together as if they were pieces of fabric. This is done through the art of stitching one topic to the next to create a conversation.

When quilting a conversation, keep an open mind about where the conversation will go, rather than having a pre-determined destination for the conversation. The most important goals of conversation quilting are to prolong the conversation and engage each participant. Each participant should contribute to the fabric of the conversation by connecting with what others say and sharing their own thoughts and experiences. Sharing information is a form of social bonding that encourages self-expression, self-awareness, memory recall, and the creation of new memories. By connecting the new experience of the conversation to long-term, hardwired foundational memories, new memories are more successfully formed.

You can quilt a conversation about any topic. Let's use the example of one of America's most loved sports: baseball. This lighthearted subject might bring back memories of vitality and the splendor of the spring and summer seasons. Start by asking the individual or group the simple question, "Do you like baseball?" Keep the conversation going by asking a follow-up question, such as, "Why not?" or, "Do you have a favorite team?" Allow each response to lead the conversation wherever it may go, and gradually stitch together a related topic, such as, "What songs are sung at baseball games?" Take the time to sing each song together. You've now combined memory and emotional learning with a new and enjoyable social experience.

CHAPTER FIFTEEN

Music as Medicine

"The power of music to integrate and cure is quite fundamental. It is the profoundest nonchemical medication."

Oliver Sacks, *Awakenings*

The use of music as medicine can promote socialization and lessen challenging behaviors such as Sundowning, which is a psychological phenomenon in which increased confusion and restlessness is experienced at the end of the day and during the night. Together with 45 residents of a memory care community, 35 of whom suffered from the symptoms of Sundowning, we embarked on an experiment which consisted of 6 months of using music as medicine. The Music as Medicine model involves choosing appropriate music to be played for the group during different times of each day. In our experiments, the Music as Medicine model resulted in a decrease of the number of participants who experienced Sundowning, reducing the number from 35 to 9 people. You can recreate this project by playing music in the living environment every day and paying special attention to three unique stages of the day which dictate the kind of music to play.

The 3-Stage Cycle of Music as Medicine

In the Music as Medicine model, Stage 1 of the cycle takes place each morning. Upbeat, popular, instrumental music with a melody is played. Take the preferences, ages, and ethnicities of participants into account, and vary musical selections so that everyone has an opportunity for maximum engagement with the music. In our study, participants could easily process the music and many could sing along with ease. Engaging with music increases serotonin and causes feelings of happiness and well-being. The morning, Stage 1, is an important stage of the day because it sets the tone for the rest of the day. The morning is like the first domino that is pushed over onto a long line of standing dominoes, each falling in turn. A successful start causes a ripple effect that results in better mood and behavior throughout the day.

Stage 2 of the process starts in the late morning or at lunch time. Play upbeat but not well-known instrumental music. This music serves as pleasant background noise that allows the brain to benefit from an increased production of serotonin but does not detract from social engagement. Music at this stage of the day increases a sense of ease in the body but does not over-stimulate or distract the mind from activities, conversation, or attentiveness to eating at mealtimes. Music with lyrics or a lyrical melody is not recommended at mealtimes because lyrics and lyrical melodies may encourage people to sing along while eating, which can cause choking.

Stage 3 of the cycle takes place in the evenings around the time when the sun is setting. This is a wonderful time to play music with one line of melody, which causes the brain to release dopamine. Dopamine relaxes the mind and body. The evening is a time of day when the brain is best suited for those mindless but necessary tasks of daily life, such as sorting and folding laundry. Performing these tasks presents an opportunity for us to engage in mindfulness.[9] We don't need to think very much about the task of sorting laundry, so it's a perfect opportunity to pay attention to our breathing, our surroundings, and the soothing music that is playing. Using this stage of the day as a meditative one has many healing benefits for both patients and caregivers.

Melodic Intonation Therapy

Melodic Intonation Therapy (MIT) is a form of speech therapy, which uses simple melodies to help those who have difficulty communicating through speech. This music-based therapy encourages the brain's right hemisphere to compensate for impaired speech abilities that are usually based in the left

---

[9] Mindfulness is further described in Chapter 16, Mindfulness for Caregivers.

hemisphere. MIT bypasses that part of the brain and returns the power of speech to some individuals who have had difficulty or inability speaking. Try MIT by taking a very familiar song and changing the lyrics to words that can be used in everyday speech. Choose a simple song with enough repetition for the brain to store the new information. Here's an example that uses the *Happy Birthday* song to help someone relearn how to say *Good Morning*.

Sing the melody of Happy Birthday and substitute the words as follows, with the original lyrics in bold and the new lyrics in italics:

Happy birthday to you
Good morning to you
Happy birthday to you
Good morning to you
Happy birthday dear Annie
Good morning everybody
Happy birthday to you
Good morning to you

MIT is an extremely useful tool for helping those with memory impairment and aphasia to regain speech. The melody of Happy Birthday is a long-term, hardwired memory that can serve as a platform for new information development. It enables the individual to bypass parts of the brain that complicate speech. With repetition, MIT invokes the power of Procedural Learning to develop and maintain the new phrases, as in the following example.

Mr. Smith had not spoken for a year when we began to use MIT to help him regain his speech. Music gave us a way to help him communicate. After three weeks of MIT, Mr. Smith developed enough ability to speak in song at his granddaughter's wedding ceremony. Through MIT, Mr. Smith got the chance to tell his granddaughter that he loved her and he wished the couple good luck. He achieved this by using the melody of My Country Tis' of Thee, replaced with new lyrics: *"I love you very much, and I wish you good luck."*

My country 'tis of thee, sweet land of liberty
I love you very much, and I wish you good luck

Music is just one form of expressive therapy that can be beneficial to those with dementia. Art, dance, poetry writing, and many other forms of expression tap into areas of the brain that enrich our connection to ourselves and each other. Expressive arts give us a way to share our inner world with others, which is especially important for those who struggle to communicate verbally. Music is often called the universal language, and the same power to invoke emotion, increase self-awareness, and unite people can apply to many other expressive arts.

CHAPTER SIXTEEN

Mindfulness for Caregivers

As the number of people living with some form of dementia is expected to triple, so too must the number of caregivers. If we hope to develop and retain talented, caring professionals in this necessary field, we must protect their health and wellbeing by exploring more stress-management and stress-reduction techniques for caregivers.

Mindfulness is a mental state of being calm, conscious, and aware of the present moment. It is achieved by focusing on one's experience of the present moment and avoiding mind-wandering, rather than being consumed by the brain's incessant judgments. You can achieve a mindful mental state at any time, during any activity, by focusing completely on the task at hand, on each and every breath that enters and exits your body, and by paying attention to the atmosphere around you.

The rhythmic repetition of our breath keeps us continuously grounded in the present moment. Focusing on our breathing brings our attention to our bodies instead of focusing solely on our thoughts. As we increase our awareness of the sensations within our bodies, we can separate ourselves from the thoughts that consistently race through our minds. The practice of mindfulness can help caregivers remain calm and centered during stressful emergencies, challenging encounters, and the day-to-day practice of connecting with the individuals for whom we care.

Mindfulness enables us to gain more control of our natural stress responses and to calm our bodies and minds. I have conducted research projects in multiple dementia care communities that have shown the benefits of mindfulness for caregivers. These research projects have consisted of two groups: Test Group A is taught mindfulness techniques, and Test Group B is given additional paid time off from work. In one such research project, members of both Test Group A and Test Group B included Certified Nursing Assistants (CNAs) and family caregivers. Participants of both test groups were randomly selected, and each consisted of five senior-level CNAs, one junior-level CNA, and one family caregiver. Group members came from all walks of life and places of origin. This experiment was conducted over a one-week period of five working days for each CNA and family caregiver.

Test Group A was selected to engage in a number of mindfulness practices. This group engaged in exercises such as mindful breathing, mindful eating, and mindful walks. They were generally encouraged to try to keep their thoughts focused on the present moment as much as possible. They engaged in mindful care through practices such as meeting patients where they are emotionally and prompting patients to focus on their present experiences and surroundings. At the end of each day, this group engaged in a ten-minute body scan and meditation session, in which they were guided to bring their attention to the relaxation of each part of their bodies while focusing on each breath.

Meanwhile, Test Group B was provided with no mindfulness instruction or guidance. Test Group B was permitted to leave thirty minutes early every day that week without any reduction in pay.

Toward the end of each CNA's work day, we conducted an end-of-day debriefing to collect feedback about their day. With family caregivers, we conducted an end-of-day phone call consisting of the same few debriefing questions. As early as day three, results showed that Test Group A was benefitting from the practice of mindfulness. The group made many positive comments about their enjoyment of the mindfulness tasks. They reported better mood, better relationships among their peers, and a better sense of awareness of their surroundings. They experienced more moments of revelation about better ways to accomplish care, from recognizing the benefit of singing a song with a patient or having a conversation to learn more about the patient. The patients that were cared for by this group exhibited fewer incidences of challenging behavior, as evidenced by behavioral logs that were kept for each group.

In addition to daily debriefing questionnaires, each caregiver also completed one five-minute feedback survey at the end of the week. The positive feedback provided by Test Group A, in combination with the positive behavior of the people for whom they provided care, shows that even in a short time, the practice of mindfulness can have a significant impact on both patient and caregiver.

Although Test Group B was allowed to leave work thirty minutes early every day, Test Group A provided more positive feedback about the week, such as increased appreciation of the important work they do and an increased sense of purpose and control. This shows that having more free time away from work is not necessarily the best way to reduce stress for dementia caregivers; however, how one spends one's free time does matter. If caregivers engage in mindfulness practices outside of work, they could likely see similar positive results.

To expand this short-term research project, I continued to collect data for a second week. Interestingly, three of the six associates from Test Group B called out of work the following week, but all of the associates from Test Group A reported to work.

One of the many benefits of mindfulness is the ripple effect that it can create. One CNA commented that she loved doing the daily mindfulness exercises so much that she brought the principles home to share with her children. A family caregiver, who takes care of her father, commented that she had been feeling overwhelmed, but practicing daily mindfulness made her feel more appreciative of the time she gets to share with her father. Research shows that stress can be a factor in developing Alzheimer's disease and many related dementias. Mindfulness can help to alleviate stress and, thus, it is a neuroprotective behavior with many health benefits.

It was eye-opening for me to see how many caregivers embraced the mindfulness approach in such a short time and with such success. CNAs are truly the backbone of the industry and their jobs are emotionally and physically demanding, yet the industry often does not provide them with the resources or tools to help them maintain their own health. Increased education and awareness about the benefits of mindfulness in dementia care can decrease the turnover rate in this industry and improve quality of life for caregivers.

Improved quality of life for caregivers also improves the quality of life for each person for whom we provide care. When we bring more mindfulness into our daily lives, we find ourselves sharing these principles with those around us. When we go for a mindful walk with a person with dementia, we point out the sound of the birds chirping, the wind through the leaves, the feeling of the sun on our faces and the ground beneath our feet. When we assist someone with dementia at mealtimes, we encourage them to enjoy the smell, color, taste, and sensation of their food, which increases appetite and can even improve digestion. Mindfulness reduces challenging behavior in people with dementia, because it improves memory and concentration while reducing agitation and stress. Try being mindful of your breath and calmly accepting the present moment. The benefit is immediate and the more you practice, the more you will see the benefits increase.

Part 3: ENGAGE

*Understanding and connection enables us
to lead engaged and productive lives.*

CHAPTER SEVENTEEN

Benefits of Engagement

While we wait for a cure, we can treat dementia through the best medicine there is: engagement with life. This can be done in both informal and professional care settings by using everyday life skills and standard clinical tactics alike. When it comes to engagement, it's not always about what we do but, rather, how we do it.

There are many positive effects of supportive living and care environments. When people with dementia are treated as the valuable individuals they are, they become empowered to courageously engage with the world around them. In a research project that I conducted with 28 residents of a Memory Support Assisted Living community, I observed profound examples of this fact. Together we embarked on an experiment in harnessing the power of music, social engagement, and performance to improve individual outcomes.

Of the residents who participated in this project, 25 had Alzheimer's disease or a related dementia. We rehearsed the singing of the Star Spangled Banner every day for 35 days. We then made an arrangement to perform the song for the community alongside the Southeastern Massachusetts Festival Chorus. When the choral group and the residents combined, they totaled more than one hundred singers. When they performed together, you could not distinguish the individuals with dementia from the rest of the group. They were just a choir of singers, singing together in unison and harmony. This experience was tremendously rewarding for the entire community and evidence of the fact that when individuals are given the opportunity, they can rise to the level of greatness that surrounds them.

As a contractor for living communities, I have often suggested that residents be given some control in making decisions for the community. Residents should be involved in selecting their activities, the music they listen to, the artwork that is displayed on the walls, and even the staff members who care for them. Under the right circumstances, it is amazing to see how people flourish when given an opportunity for this kind of authoritative engagement. For example, at a Memory Support community that was having difficulty with associate retention, we created a resident hiring committee. The residents reviewed each application and took part in the interview process. I conducted the initial interview, then invited each resident to come and ask a few prepared questions. This system was successful, and we hired the most impressive applicants. Months later, the retention rate for new associates had improved drastically.

When we provide interesting and engaging experiences for people with dementia, we create an environment in which they can sustain their skills for longer, and within which they can put their skills to meaningful use. Now that we recognize the importance of neuroplasticity and how we can help promote it, we know that being actively engaged in one's life reinforces the memory and can strengthen and bypass damaged parts of the brain. These results are concrete and measurable.

In another research project, I measured the daily engagement levels of thirty residents through mini-mental exams, which are standard thirty-point questionnaires that are commonly used in clinical settings to assess cognitive impairment. I recorded each resident's performance on the exams over a period of six months. The residents who engaged in the cognitive challenges of these mini-mental exams increased their cognitive capacity from moderate memory loss, to having almost no signs or symptoms of memory loss. One resident developed enough sustainable engagement that she was able to move home from the care facility and is now living independently with the support of her family. She and I continue to meet for lunch regularly.

Remember, in dementia care, it's not always about what you do; sometimes how you do it is what matters. You can increase the benefits of engagement by reframing everyday tasks. Turn getting dressed into an engaging activity by helping the person to select his or her own clothes every day. Give cues and two options, such as, "Mr. Smith, would you like to wear this black sweater or this blue shirt tomorrow?" Lay out each article of clothing in the order in which they will be put on.

Turn bathing into an engaging activity by talking through the process and offering a loofa to hold onto. Holding an object helps someone with cognitive impairment to focus their energy, and it limits flailing and hitting that can sometimes be the reaction to the feeling of water against their skin. A loofa also provides a dignified way for them to feel that they are washing themselves even if they are not.

Turn dining into an engaging activity by making sure the meal is easy to eat and captures their attention. Use red plates to stimulate the appetite of someone who doesn't each much. For those who have difficulty using utensils, try baking the meal in a muffin tray to create a single-serving portion. Instead of serving steak, potato, and vegetable, provide support by baking individual portions of ground meat and soft-cooked or pureed vegetables in a muffin tin.

You can also use culinary puree molds to form pureed food into recognizable shapes. Mold pureed carrots into the shape of whole carrots or pureed meat into the shape of a steak. These methods keep mealtimes fun and manageable. When frustration is decreased, engagement is increased. Dining scarves are another way to improve mealtimes; use them to create a protective layer that keeps clothes clean and helps signify the beginning and the end of the meal.

CHAPTER EIGHTEEN

Engaging Through Color

The psychology of color is widely recognized as the impact that color has on us. Color can influence our behavior, mood, and attention so powerfully that color choices are used deliberately to influence us in a variety of ways, from the intentional use of color in present day marketing material to the ancient Chinese art of Feng Shui. Harness the power of color in your approach to care by using specific colors during different activities and throughout the individual's living environment.

Here are some basic tips:
- Use color to provide contrast in spaces. Dementia makes all-white rooms difficult to navigate.
- Use a colored toilet set to ensure contrast and direct attention.

- Choose different colors for sheets, blankets, and pillowcases. White sheets and blankets can be difficult to distinguish from one another.
- Dark and bright shades of all colors can be hard to see. When in doubt, choose a medium-shade.

You can use different colors to promote different behaviors.

Red:
- Red plates and cups can increase appetite and encourage a person with memory impairment to eat more. Red plates also provide contrast between the food and the plate.
- Painting a bedroom door red makes the door easier to distinguish from the wall, whereas a white door within a white wall can be difficult to find. Painting the inside of a bedroom door red may encourage someone to come out of their room more often.
- Red promotes participation. Think of ways you can use red to meet various individual goals, such as using red shoes to encourage walking, a red ball to improve focus during a game of catch, or red-based jigsaw puzzles to promote cognitive skills.
- Avoid wearing red when visiting a loved one because it can also be perceived as an intimidating color.
- Don't mistake orange for red:

o Orange increases stagnant focus, meaning it draws attention but does not foster participation.

Green:

- Green can increase reading ability through neurological sequencing and subconscious conditioning: we are conditioned to associate green with "go" which makes text that is written in green font easier for the brain to follow.[10]

- Green can stimulate energy while also promoting relaxation.

- Green is a great color for caregivers to wear because it is often the last color we lose the ability to see. A consistent caregiver uniform or shirt can also help individuals to identify their caregivers.

- Try putting green tape on the handle of objects, such as walkers, if you notice someone frequently reaching for that object and having difficulty finding it.

- Green is a great color to wear when visiting your loved one because it fosters engagement, relaxation, and peace.

---

[10] This research was derived from reading exercises with residents of a dementia care community. I printed copies of reading material in green, blue, and pink and observed that participants read faster, with better reading comprehension and fewer misread words when the text is printed in green. I tracked these results through a simple tally system alongside reading comprehension questions.

Purple:

- Purple can stimulate imagination and spirituality.
- Purple is the color of royalty, and we subconsciously perceive purple objects as valuable or expensive.
- Choose purple to encourage someone to think of an object as sacred and desirable, such as when providing them with a personal journal.

Yellow:

- Yellow increases feelings of happiness.
- We tend to associate yellow with sunshine.
- In my observation, people tend to smile more in yellow rooms.
- People with dementia tend to wander into yellow rooms and stay there for longer periods of time, which is why common rooms that are intended for social interaction in residential care facilities are often painted yellow.

Blue:

- Blue promotes a relaxed mood.
- Painting a room blue can decrease confusion and increase concentration.
- Blue is great color to wear for a visit with your loved one because it reassures them that you are not a threat.

White:

- White is difficult to see. An all-white room can appear circular to someone with dementia. Provide contrast by painting one or two accent walls, or creating other colorful focal points within the room.

- It can be difficult for someone with dementia to distinguish between white blankets and sheets. Provide contrasting color by choosing different colors for blankets, pillowcases, and sheets.

- Avoid white plates in favor of red plates. Many foods will be easier to see on a red plate than on a white plate.

- People with dementia sometimes have trouble finding the toilet seat because bathrooms are often all white. It can be very helpful to install a toilet seat in a contrasting color such as black or dark green.

Black:

- Black is often associated with frightening thoughts and mourning.

- Black can prevent communication and increase separation among people.

- Avoid using black welcome mats or carpets. A black welcome mat might be perceived as hole which people with dementia might refuse to cross or attempt to tip-toe around.

- Black can also be interpreted as a color of power and control that protects the wearer from feeling overly exposed or vulnerable.

Experiment with the intentional use of specific colors throughout the home or living environment. Observe how different colors can affect individual performance during daily activities. Some people are more receptive to, and aware of, the impact of color on mood than others, but the power of color to provide visual contrast is undisputed. Color directs attention and helps the eye distinguish different objects, which can have tremendous benefits for those with cognitive and visual impairments.

CHAPTER NINETEEN

Structure and Routine

Structure and routine are important for people with memory impairment and dementia. The greater the individual's sense of routine, the greater the chance that he or she will look forward to activities and experience success in repeated engagement with them. Daily routines empower successful outcomes. When daily activities become familiar, they're more likely to be performed well. Successful outcomes increase the likelihood of participation. In turn, the social interaction and sense of accomplishment that comes with participation in daily activities increases mental health and happiness.

For people with dementia, consistent daily routines have been proven to increase engagement, help sustain life skills for longer, and decrease isolation and apathy. Since coping with change can be challenging, a structured routine can help maintain a sense of stability. A living environment with a structured routine is a supportive environment because it reinforces a sense of normalcy and familiarity. This leads to less agitation and easier transitions between daily activities.

Routines also validate a sense of purpose in a dignified way. When we all have daily routines within a community, our roles are easier to recognize and normalize. Someone with dementia might need help to complete their routine, and our consistency as caregivers continuously reinforces that we are there to help them every day.

The following is a sample schedule that uses the Activities of Daily Living, the Four Dimensions of Sustainability, and Music as Medicine to optimize productivity and positivity throughout the day. Remember that different people have different preferences, and may require more or less time to complete certain activities. Use this schedule as a general guide and modify it as necessary for the individual.

Time	Activity	Music
6:45am	Alarm	Upbeat, popular, instrumental music with a lyrical melody
7:00am	Quiet morning activity: watch the news in bed, review the schedule for the day ahead, make the bed, water the plants	
7:15am	Get ready for the day: bathe, brush teeth, wash face, get dressed	
8:00am	Help prepare breakfast and set the table	

8:30am	Eat breakfast	Instrumental
9:00am	Clean up after breakfast	Upbeat, popular, instrumental music with a lyrical melody
9:30am	Physical activity: go for a walk, participate in light stretching, physical therapy, or group exercise	
10:30am	Emotional activity: attend a spiritual service (in person, on the radio, or on television), visit with family or friends	
11:30am	Social activity: continued social visit, participate in a conversation or activity, help prepare lunch	
12:30pm	Eat lunch	Instrumental
1:00pm	Clean up after lunch	Upbeat popular music without lyrics
1:30pm	Free time for activities, quiet reflection, organizational projects, social interaction, errands, or appointments	
4:30pm	Help prepare dinner	
5:00pm	Eat dinner	Instrumental
5:30pm	Help clean up after dinner	Soothing, relaxing music
6:00pm	Cognitive activity: Bingo, board game, jigsaw puzzle, or crafts project	
7:00pm	Evening movie, television show, book, or magazine with herbal tea or decaffeinated coffee	
8:30pm	Get ready for bed: wash face, brush teeth, put on pajamas, write three good things that happened that day in an Appreciation Journal	

Recording three positive events daily, aloud or in a journal, is an easy way to activate Cognitive Restructuring. Cognitive Restructuring is a therapeutic process that anyone can use to shift our perspective from negative and irrational, to positive and hopeful. Taking time to focus on three positive events that happened each day keeps us on the lookout for good things, and helps us to see that our lives are filled with blessings and benefits.

CHAPTER TWENTY

Understanding Behaviors

In dementia care, the term "behavior" is often used to describe a specific negative or concerning action exhibited by a patient. This is a term of which we as caregivers should be wary. It shows a lack of compassionate understanding in our interpretation of the actions of those for whom we care. No one simply has behaviors. Everyone has needs. Typically, a concerning behavior occurs when a human need is not being met. The person is likely not just acting out for the sake of making your job more difficult. Their behavior may simply be an expression that the person:

- Needs to use the bathroom
- Feels lost, confused, or overwhelmed
- Feels frustrated by an inability to verbally communicate

Changing our perception of people's behaviors enables us to be better detectives in our mission to identify and fulfill the needs of others.

The following is an example of how it is possible to leverage a need behavior to create a positive outcome for the individual and the community. Mrs. Smith was in the mid-stages of dementia. Every morning, she exhibited a need behavior by yelling at her caregiver. She would wrap herself in her blankets and say that her house had been broken into. Everyone said, "Mrs. Smith has dementia; she's just making it up." They ignored her behavior. After talking with Mrs. Smith for few minutes, we noticed that some of what she was saying had truth behind it. We discovered that the night shift was completing their room checks by opening her door and shining a flashlight in to make sure everyone was safely in bed. Mrs. Smith interpreted this as someone breaking in. Her behavior reflected a need for explanation, reassurance, and a sense of safety. In response to our increased understanding of Mrs. Smith's perspective, we explained the situation to her and ensured that future room checks were completed without a flashlight. Mrs. Smith's need behavior went away.

When we think of the people for whom we care as unique individuals with valid viewpoints, we realize that in most cases, there is truth behind what they say. People may express their feelings in ways that do not make their true feelings immediately clear to us, but if we genuinely want to help, we must take the time to try to understand.

If a person with dementia develops a negative habit, such as stealing objects from around the house or community, why not leverage that behavior to increase their engagement? Create some rummaging space in the top drawer of a dresser where they can store everything they hoard. Through Procedural Learning, a person with dementia can learn to put these objects into the drawer routinely in an average of 35 days. Ultimately, with a caregiver's reminders, the person will likely become consistent about putting the things they hoard into this determined place. Then, when things go missing, you'll know where to retrieve them.

Brimming is another type of need behavior that is often classified as negative. Brimming is a term that refers to repetitive expressions, whether verbal or physical, such as clicking a pen repeatedly or tapping our fingers on a table. Verbally, we often hear repetitive questions or words such as, "Help, help" or, "I'm hungry, I'm hungry." Both physical and verbal brimming can be leveraged to become a tool for increased engagement. For example, repetitive tapping can be leveraged into engagement with music. You will notice that if you play a person's preferred music (which is usually music that the person listened to from age 18 to 25) their habit of tapping can become very therapeutic for them and less agitating to others. For those who repetitively say the same thing over and over, try to engage them to sing a well-known song with a repetitive chorus, such as "Sweet Chariot." Singing a repetitive chorus may bypass the part of the brain which feels compelled to say "Help" when they replace "Help" with the words to a beautiful song.

In one residential community, I worked with a woman who would repeatedly yell, "Help, help!" It was disturbing for many visitors, and it led to a lot of complaints. I decided to do some Reflective

Behavior Trending (RBT) with her. RBT is the repetition of a desired behavior after a non-desired behavior has occurred. In this case, every time she yelled "Help, help," I would whisper "Hello, welcome." After doing this three times a week for five weeks, this woman replaced "Help, help!" with a soft, "Hello, welcome." She became part of the community's welcoming committee.

Next time you see behavior that is in need of modification, don't focus on how much it's driving you crazy; think of it as an opportunity to leverage the behavior in a way that will engage that person to be a happier member of the community.

More tips:
- Gather detailed information about the person's preferences and personality. This will come in handy when helping to redirect the person to more positive behavior.
- Document challenging behaviors in detail. Make note of what time of day the behavior is exhibited.
- Be aware of your own attitudes and feelings in response to challenging behavior. Calm promotes calm; agitation promotes agitation.

CHAPTER TWENTY-ONE

Inappropriate Sexual Behavior

Not all sexual acts are meant to be sexual. Sometimes it is context that makes the behavior inappropriate. Before making a judgement, consider the fact that someone with dementia may not be able to adequately assess their surroundings; thus, they may not intend for an otherwise normal behavior to be inappropriate. For example, masturbation is inappropriate in public, but someone with dementia might not make that connection.

The use of sexual language can be the result of an emotional outburst that is caused by dementia. Inappropriately touching others might be caused by nonsexual attention-seeking. Try to understand the behavior and what it is communicating. Could it be driven by loneliness? Lack of engagement? Confusion? Look for causes that might underlie the action, and don't assume that the intention is always sexual.

How to react

Don't ignore the behavior. If it is notable or persistent, talk about it with a doctor or care professional. Inappropriate behavior of a sexual nature can be caused by an issue that is related to acute illness or medication. Try not to get upset or offended if someone speaks to you inappropriately. Respond calmly; for example, "I understand that you want to say that, but it hurts my feelings and makes me uncomfortable." Calmly assert your boundaries by attempting to redirect the individual to another subject or conversation, or offer an appropriate object to hold, such as a comforting pillow.

Regard inappropriate behavior as a symptom of the person's condition. People with dementia sometimes do not have a filter for what is socially appropriate; they sometimes say and do the first thing that comes into their mind. Scolding someone with dementia by telling them that their behavior is inappropriate will not help. If they understood that it was inappropriate, they would not do it to begin with. When approaching someone who is behaving in a sexually inappropriate manner, introduce yourself. This supplies the person with a reminder of the nature of your relationship. When they realize that you are a caregiver, they will understand that you are a professional who is there to help them rather than someone who is there for companionship. This may help clarify the context of the interaction, and they may naturally correct their behavior.

Don't give mixed messages. Hand-holding, hugs, and kisses can be confusing. Use discretion and err on the conservative side. Wear appropriate clothing. Be aware of your own attitudes and feelings.

It can be helpful to document inappropriate behavior in detail by using a behavioral log. Try to evaluate whether the behavior is happening at specific locations, times of day, around certain individuals, or in response to specific potential triggers. Detailed information about the behavior comes in handy when helping to redirect the person. Work with fellow members of the community to individualize care approaches.

A behavioral log can be used to document inappropriate or concerning behavior of any kind:

Date	Time	Behavior	Location	Individuals present	Possible triggers

Recognize triggers:
- Sexually explicit material in the environment
- Observing personal care given to someone of opposite sex
- Seeing someone of the opposite sex in bed
- Underwear on backwards
- Loose fanny pack
- Provocative, inappropriate, or tight clothing
- Loneliness and lack of engagement
- Certain substances can also cause sexual side effects, including alcohol and dopamine agonists.

CHAPTER TWENTY-TWO

Wandering

Engagement is not only good for the brain and the spirit, but it is also associated with a drastic decrease in the incidence of wandering. There are two different types of wandering: Random Wandering and Goal-Driven Wandering. Whether the person is inclined to wander randomly without a purpose, or if they tend to wander with a goal in mind, such as a stated desire to get to a particular location, they are less are apt to wander if they are more engaged with the activities of their daily life.

Increase engagement to decrease wandering. Invite individuals to help with tasks around the house or community. Provide a rummaging box filled with objects they love or activities they love to do. This can include simple household objects, such as a silverware organizer in which they can match up all of the silverware into the correct location, a box full of photos or a photo album, or a themed rummaging box containing small objects in any theme that the person prefers whether it be fishing, cars, gardening, or animals.

People with dementia tend to wander in the direction of their dominant hand. This can be important to know if someone walks outside unaccompanied. If they are right-handed, they may have gone right; if they are left-handed, they may have gone left.

Paint exit doors the same color as the walls in the room. If the room is white, painting the exit door white will keep their focus off of the exit. Bright colors, particularly red, increases focus on objects. When the inside of an exit door is red, people with dementia may feel encouraged to open the door and walk out. This can be beneficial when encouraging someone to venture out of their bedroom, yet it can increase the potential for danger if it encourages someone to walk out the front door and onto the street.

Put notes on the door that say, "I will be back soon," even if you are just upstairs. A person with memory impairment may forget that you are upstairs and decide to wander out of the house.

Remove coats, umbrellas, and shoes from plain view. These objects can trigger people with dementia to wander outside. If you are visiting someone in a residential community, try to avoid wearing a jacket during your visit because it can trigger your loved one to want to go home.

To be prepared in the event that someone with dementia does wander away alone, it is helpful to create a one-page fact sheet that includes the person's name, nickname, a recent color photo and physical description, information about the person's favorite activities, and where they might be found. Some brief background information, or a prepared question to ask the person can be helpful tools to direct the person back home. Help a police officer or neighbor to approach the person with a comforting statement, such as, "Betty is making chicken tonight; it's time to go home for dinner." Keep a few copies of this fact sheet in your car, home, vacation home, and on your person because if you ever need it, you will be relieved to have it handy.

Many organizations can provide help for individuals with dementia who are at risk for wandering. Consider registering for a program such as MedicAlert + Alzheimer's Association Safe Return,[11] which is a 24-hour, nationwide emergency response service for individuals who tend to wander or are at risk for other medical emergencies.

---

[11] More information about this service can be found on the Alzheimer's Association website, and the MedicAlert Foundation website.

CHAPTER TWENTY-THREE

Adapting to Change

We all change over time. Some changes we make by choice, and some changes are out of our control. Big changes that are out of our control can be very difficult to cope with, but for our well-being, we must learn to adapt.

Some of the changes that accompany dementia can be sad and scary. We must try to be hopeful and vigilant in our pursuit of happiness. The key to successfully maintaining a high quality of life throughout the progression of dementia is acceptance and engagement. Whether it is engaging with the Activities of Daily Living, communication with others, or the love of nature, food, or music, focus on abilities instead of inabilities. Work to understand the perspective of the person for whom you care, and strive to provide the right level of support.

The best way to support someone throughout the changes that accompany dementia is to focus on what they are able to do at that moment rather than worrying about what they used to be able to do in the past. Try not to focus on the tasks they cannot complete, even if they were able to do something yesterday that they cannot do today.

Focusing on the person as they are in the present moment is a form of genuine understanding and compassion. Throughout the progression of dementia, skills may come and go depending on what the person is experiencing at that moment. Maintaining a focus on the present moment is a key element of mindfulness that will improve your interactions with those around you.

When you focus on the present, rather than clinging to the past, you approach each moment with an optimism that creates space for good things to happen. This doesn't mean that good things will always happen, but it does mean that we won't overlook the simple and successful moments that we might not otherwise notice if we are too busy thinking about the past. We should celebrate each moment of happiness with those who are in our care. Our presence can encourage them to continue finding bountiful blessings in their lives even though they are adapting to a new life with dementia.

CHAPTER TWENTY-FOUR

Visiting a Loved One

A visit from a loved one might be a special and meaningful part of the day for a person with dementia. This chapter is primarily for those who have a friend or family member with dementia. Professional caregivers can share the information in this chapter with friends and family members of residents to improve their visits. Here are some ways to ensure that visits go as smoothly as possible:

- Plan visits at a time of day that is best for your loved one's schedule. Morning and afternoon visits are preferable to evening visits because people generally experience more confusion in the evening.
- Bring something special to share, such as a favorite song to play, a book to read, or a photo album. A cherished object can be a useful tool for increasing socialization and participation.

- Small groups of one, two, or three visitors are ideal. They enable more genuine connection and can be less overwhelming.
- Large groups and social events might be manageable. Try to partake in events and community activities that do not require excessive physical activity or over-stimulating atmospheres. You and your loved one must both feel at ease.
- Avoid wearing outerwear during visits with people who cannot leave a residential care community. A coat, hat, gloves, or even a pocketbook can be emotional triggers that cause your loved one to want to go home.
- Parting at the end of a visit can be emotionally difficult. Try to keep your mood as positive as possible. Do what you can to help them transition into their next activity.

As dementia progresses, you will notice changes in people's ability to communicate verbally due to cognitive challenges. Trouble finding words, increased confusion, and even inappropriate behavior are all normal. Remember to keep conversation simple, and initiate it by introducing yourself at the beginning of your visit. A simple, "Hi, Mom; it's your son, Jimmy," can be very helpful. Speak slowly, and ask one question at a time. Give your loved one time to answer the question. If they do not respond, try again. If they continue to be unresponsive, try a different subject or introduce an activity.

Body language is an important tool for communication especially as dementia progresses. What emotions do you sense behind their words and actions? What sense are you conveying to them with your physical behavior? How can you use your posture and vocal tone to make the interaction more pleasant, calming, and clear? Encourage non-verbal communication through pointing or gesturing when someone has difficulty expressing themselves or recalling a word. Maintain good eye contact so that you do not overlook non-verbal communication.

Be aware of your own feelings during the visit. If you are getting irritated, tense, or feeling rushed, it may confuse or upset someone with dementia. Take a deep breath and try to relax. Take breaks when you need them. Feelings of irritability are a clue that your mind needs time to refresh.

Setting up Successful Transitions

Conversations should have a clear start and a clear end as should interactions and activities. Introduce yourself and state your intention:

- *Hi, Mom; it's Josh. I'm here to visit you!*
- *Hello, Mrs. Smith; I'm Angela, and I'm here to help you with your shower today.*
- *Good morning, Phil; it's your wife, Ellen. You look handsome today! Would you like to go out to lunch with me?*
- *Good afternoon, folks; I'm Chris, and I'm here to lead you in a fun group activity.*

At the end of the interaction or activity, connect with each person by offering them a handshake or a hug and verbally thanking them for their participation.

Positive and forward-thinking statements at the end of visits can ease the transition of your departure. Say things like, "I enjoyed our visit, and I hope you enjoyed it, too," or, "Maybe next time we can go out for ice cream." Help to guide them through the transition by knowing their schedule and giving them a reminder such as, "It's time for you to eat dinner, but I'll see you again tomorrow."

CHAPTER TWENTY-FIVE

Handling the Holidays

The stress of the holidays can take a toll on families, so make sure to plan ahead. Invite family and friends to meet as a group before the event. Discuss location, transportation plans, the menu, and activities to do during the event. Decide which traditions you might need to adapt and which you would like to keep the same. Handling the holidays with a family member who has dementia is easier if everyone provides some level of support so that special considerations are not planned and facilitated all by one person. If you are the primary family caregiver of someone with dementia, make sure you communicate with others and ask them for help when you need it.

Keep it Familiar

For many people, a change in schedule and environment (even a visit home or to a loved one's home) can cause anxiety and confusion. If you are planning to take your loved one home from a residential community, try to show up early and spend some time with them first before inviting them to come home with you. This will provide a smoother transition, and it allows them to process the information at their own speed. Carefully consider whether bringing your loved one to an unfamiliar or forgotten environment will be worth the risks. In some cases, it may be wise to hold a small family celebration in their residential community instead. Attempt to plan your visit and your celebration around their schedule as much as possible. Sticking to their routine will greatly improve their chances of success.

Keep it Small and Simple

Plan for small groups of friends or family members to arrive to the celebration at staggered times. Even if your loved one is not sure who they are, two or three new faces are likely to be welcome while a large group of people might be overwhelming. Remember to introduce each person. Encourage each person to also introduce themselves and give a compliment: "Happy Thanksgiving, Aunt Mary! I'm your nephew, John. I'm happy to see you today!"

Consider Time and Place

People with dementia often get tired easily, especially as their condition declines. Knowing that confusion is more common in the evening, try to schedule your event or visit in the morning or midday, which are the times of day least associated with confusion. If you decide to hold an evening event, ensure that the area is well lit, and avoid anything that may trigger a need behavior. The trigger may be a visit to his or her old bedroom or bringing up the death of a sibling or friend. Be sensitive of feelings, and keep interactions positive.

Respect Traditions and Memories

Focus on events that are meaningful to your loved one. Things such as singing a favorite holiday song or looking at old photo albums can be very comforting for someone with dementia. Your loved one might still be able to participate by helping to mash potatoes or mix cake batter. Keep traditions alive to reinforce positive memories. If he or she always made cinnamon rolls, make cinnamon rolls together. Things such as opening holiday cards or wrapping gifts can be a great way to connect during the holidays. Rather than focusing on the result of the activity, such as creating perfectly wrapped presents, try to focus on the process instead. A feeling of connection with you is what will truly engage and comfort your loved one.

Try Not to Over-Decorate

Flashing lights and bulky decorative displays can cause disorientation and confusion. Avoid hazards such as lit candles as well as decorations that might be mistaken for edible treats, such as wax or plastic fruit, or decorative glass marbles.

Slow Down and Enjoy

Although most of us enjoy the cheerfulness of holiday music, gatherings, and meal preparation, it all adds up to noise, which can cause overstimulation. For a person with dementia, environment can be everything. Try to create an environment that is as calming as possible. Make sure they have plenty of places to relax and sit down. Schedule the day in a way that gives your loved one time to rest as well as engage with others.

CHAPTER TWENTY-SIX

Self-Care

One of the first things they say on an airplane is that if the oxygen masks come down, put on your own mask first before helping others with theirs. You cannot care for someone else before you care for yourself. The quality of care that you provide for yourself is even more important when you are responsible for another person. The healthier, stronger, and more prepared you are, the better a caregiver you will be.

Simple pleasures such as walking with a friend, reading a book, or getting a massage are very important for your peace of mind. Engaging in hobbies or joining a club or committee can help you feel a sense of accomplishment and reward for the hard work that you do. Use the mindfulness practices, described in Chapter 16, to reduce your stress and increase your resiliency to stressful moments. Use positive daily affirmations, such as, "I love what I do, and it makes a difference" to boost your spirit and create new automatic scripts in your mind.

Helpful Tips:
- Find someone, such as a friend or counselor, who can listen, give you new ideas, or simply provide a different perspective on things.
- Attend conferences and lectures about Alzheimer's disease and dementia, which will help you understand what is ahead and what resources are available.
- Make time for yourself, and make sure you use it to do the things you like to do.
- Make and keep plans with friends, family, community clubs, or take a vacation.
- Join a support group where you can make connections with people who are going through the same thing as you are.
- Consider enrolling your loved one in an adult day care program.

Taking Time for Yourself

Take good care of your health. Eat properly, exercise, and have some "me time" to recharge your batteries. If you need a day for yourself, take it. This does not make you selfish; it allows you to refocus and build the endurance you need for the long haul. When you maintain your health, you improve the lives of those around you. You cannot help others if you if do not take care of yourself.

We often feel guilty about putting ourselves first. It is extremely important to recognize that taking care of yourself is not something to feel guilty about. Instead, you should be proud of every effort you make to promote your own health and well-being. The role of caregiver can be overwhelming, and it's okay to acknowledge this reality as a natural part of the coping process. Feeling overwhelmed is your mind and body's way of reminding you to take the best possible care of yourself.

Help and Limitations

We all need help at different times in our lives. People sometimes have trouble asking for or accepting help because they worry about being perceived as weak or a burden. Keep in mind that allowing someone else to help you can be a gift to them. It is human nature to want to help others. Don't take the role of caregiver solely upon yourself if you don't need to. Ask a trusted friend, family member, or professional caregiver to spend time with your loved one for a few hours while you do errands, groceries, or something fun. Accepting help gives others an opportunity to do something that will make them feel good, too.

It's also important to know your limits and your boundaries. Become comfortable with saying "no" to things that are too stressful for you. Give yourself permission to say things like, "Yes, I need help" or, "No, this isn't a good year for me to host a large family event."

The Mind-Body Connection

Not getting enough sleep is a major cause of illness and stress in caregivers. Without adequate sleep, you might become irritable, frustrated, or resentful. We all have limitations, so try not to push your mind or your body too hard; doing so it could lead to a burnout. Rest when you need to, and aim for eight hours of sleep each night.

Mindfulness and meditation are key tools for attaining a healthy and communicative relationship between your mind and body. Exercise can also be a powerful psychological tool to quiet external stresses and force you to focus on your internal state. Exercise has the power to combat depression and prevent a host of other health problems including dementia. Nutrition is also an important key to health that should not be overlooked. Make it a priority to eat regular, nutritious meals and snacks every day.

When I talk with family caregivers, one of their primary fears is about what will happen to their loved one if something happens to them. Worrying doesn't help. Taking excellent care of yourself does.

In the words of the poet Maya Angelou, "People will forget what you said, people will forget what you did, but people will never forget how you made them feel." *The Dementia Concept* offers tools to impact the quality of your care in a way that makes people feel valued, appreciated, and acknowledged. This, as I hope you will witness in your own care practice, can have a profound impact on individual levels of success.

With a better understanding of dementia and practical tools for how to meaningfully connect and engage with others through care, you are ready to put *The Dementia Concept* into action. The next time you are working with someone with dementia, remember these tools, which are now yours to customize into the most caring and personalized approach for each individual in your care.

Through an improved and mindful approach to interaction, conversation, expressive arts therapy, and the creation and maintenance of a regular daily schedule, you can greatly improve the life of someone with dementia. You can bring more positivity, light, and love into patient-caregiver relationships in ways that are scientifically proven to positively affect the brain. Individually, these changes might seem small, but when you put them all together, amazing things are possible.

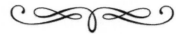

Thank you for joining the movement to improve dementia care.

May compassion, peace, and inspiration guide you on your journey.

ACKNOWLEDGEMENTS

The Dementia Concept has been years in the making, beginning with my education, through years of working directly with those affected by dementia. Thank you to my teachers and mentors for dedicating their lives, as I have, to improving the lives and the care of people with dementia. The insights we've shared have been integral to the development of this contemporary approach.

I have great appreciation for those who are living with dementia. I have been continuously amazed by how much they can still do. I'm so appreciative of all the residents and families who have shared their lives with me and trusted in my care. We have made so much progress together, and I hope what I have learned and documented in this book will help many others.

Thank you to my family, friends, and mentors. This book would not have been possible without your generosity and support. Thanks for your patience with my extreme focus on this project during all the time I have spent writing.

This book could not have been written without the work of my editor, Angela Simonelli, or the valuable feedback from our group of peer-readers. Your dedication to this book and all of your input is greatly appreciated.

Alzheimer's Association
919 North Michigan Avenue | Suite | Chicago, IL
60611-1676 | Helpline 1.800.272.3900 |
www.alz.org

**Alzheimer's Disease Education and Referral
Center (ADEAR) | National Institute on Aging**
P.O. Box 8250 | Silver Spring, MD 20907-8250
1.800.438.4380 | www.nia.nih.gov/alzheimers

Alzheimer's Foundation of America
322 Eighth Avenue | New York, NY 10001
Helpline 1.866.232.8484 | www.alzfdn.org

**Family Caregiver Alliance | National Center on
Caregiving (FCA)**
785 Market St. | Suite 750 | San Francisco, CA
94103 | 1.973-729-6601 | www.caregiver.org

Family Caregiver Network
1130 Connecticut Avenue NW | Suite 300 |
Washington, DC 20036 | 1.202.454-3970 |
www.caregiveraction.org

National Alliance for Caregiving
4720 Montgomery Lane | Suite 205 | Bethesda, MD
20814 | www.caregiving.org

**National Association of Professional Geriatric
Care Managers (GCM)**
1604 N. Country Club Road | Tucson, AZ 85716-
33102 | 1.520.881.8008 | www.aginglifecare.org

National Family Caregivers Association (NFCA)
10400 Connecticut Avenue | Suite 500 |
Kensington, MD 20895-3944 | 1.800.896.3650
www.ninds.nih.gov

National Certification Board for Alzheimer Care
3170 N Sheridan Rd | Suite 1008 | Chicago, IL
60657-4882 | www.ncbac.net

**International/National Council of Certified
Dementia Practitioners**
103 Valley View Trail | Sparta, NJ 07871
1.973-729-6601 | www.nccdp.org

International Caregivers Association
P.O. Box 193| Mapleton, ME 04757
1.207.764.1214 |
www.internationalcaregiversassociation.com

Acetylcholine: A neurotransmitter in the brain that is involved in learning and memory. Acetylcholine levels are greatly diminished in people with dementia.

Activities of daily living (ADLs): Personal care activities that are necessary for everyday life, such as eating, bathing, dressing, and using the bathroom.

Adult day services: Programs that provide opportunities for older adults to interact with others, usually in a community or dedicated center.

Advance Directive (Living Will): A document written when in good health that informs family and health care providers of one's wishes for extended medical treatment if such treatment becomes necessary.

Adverse reaction: A clinical term that includes any unexpected health or behavioral changes in reaction to a drug.

Aggression: Hitting, pushing, or threatening behavior. It is not uncommon for people with dementia to display aggression toward caregivers during assistance with daily living activities, such as grooming and dressing.

Agitation: Vocal or physical behavior, such as screaming, shouting, complaining, moaning, cursing, pacing, fidgeting, wandering, etc., which can be disruptive, unsafe, or interferes with the delivery of care.

Alternative and complementary therapies: Techniques that are used for treatment instead of, or as a complement to, drugs, surgery, or other conventional interventions. Common alternative or complementary therapies include the practice of meditation, exercise, expressive arts, reflexology, massage, and acupuncture.

Alzheimer's Disease: The most common form of dementia, which causes memory loss and damage to the hippocampus, where memories are stored.

Ambulation: The ability to walk and move freely.

Amygdala: Part of the brain located in the limbic system, which process memory through emotions.

Amyloid: An abnormal protein that the body deposits in various parts of the brain. Amyloid plaques are found in the brains of those with Alzheimer's disease.

Antidepressants, or Selective serotonin reuptake inhibitors (SSRIs): Medications that are prescribed for depression. SSRIs block a receptor in brain cells that absorbs serotonin.

Aphasia: Difficulty recalling and formulating words. Loss of language ability. Mild aphasia refers to occasional difficulty with word recall. Moderate aphasia refers to marked difficulty with word recall. Extreme aphasia refers to word recall that is limited to a few words or the complete inability to recall words.

Behaviors, challenging behaviors, and behavioral symptoms: Symptoms of dementia that are caused by difficulty processing emotions. These behaviors can include wandering, inappropriate sexual behavior, aggression, agitation, sleep disturbances, and other outward signs of depression and anxiety.

Beneficiary: An individual who is designated to receive something, such as money or property, following the death of a benefactor who has named the beneficiary in a document such as a will, trust, or insurance policy.

Binswanger's disease: A type of dementia that is associated with changes in the brain caused by stroke.

Biomarker: A marker that is used to indicate or measure a biological process such as levels of a specific protein in blood or spinal fluid. Detecting biomarkers that are specific to a disease can aid in the diagnosis and treatment of individuals with that disease as well as those who may be at risk but have not yet experienced symptoms.

Biotechnology: The use of biology (the study of living things) and biological processes to make goods or develop technologies for the benefit of humanity. Biotechnology is often used in the fields of food, drugs, and energy.

Blood-brain barrier: The selective barrier that controls the entry of substances from the blood into the brain.

Caregiver: Someone who is in charge of caring for another. A primary caregiver for those with dementia is usually a family member or a designated health care professional.

Care planning or Service plan: A written action plan that contains strategies for delivering care that addresses an individual's specific needs and challenges.

Case management: A term that is used to describe formal services that are planned by care professionals.

Cerebral cortex: The outer layer of the brain, which consists of nerve cells and the pathways that connect them. The cerebral cortex is the part of the brain in which thought processes take place. In Alzheimer's disease, nerve cells in the cerebral cortex degenerate and die.

Choline: A brain transmitter that enables cells to communicate with each other.

Clinical Social Worker (CSW): An individual who has specialized training in identifying, accessing, and assessing community resources, such as adult daycare, home care, or nursing home services, as well as individual and group counseling.

Clinical trial: A type of research study that evaluates the results of a new medical treatment, drug, or device.

Coexisting illness: A medical condition that exists simultaneously with another medical condition, such as arthritis and dementia.

Cognitive ability: Mental ability, such as judgment, memory, learning, comprehension, and reasoning.

Cognitive disorder: Psychiatric disorder that is manifested in memory deficits, altered or impaired perception, and difficulty with problem solving.

Cognitive symptom of dementia: Symptoms that relate to impaired thought processes, such as learning, comprehension, memory, reasoning and judgment.

Combativeness: Aggression or agitation.

Competence: A person's ability to make informed choices.

Continuum of care: Care services that are available to assist individuals throughout the course of a disease.

Cortical dementia: Dementia that is associated with disease that affects the cerebral cortex, causing impairments in abstract thinking, attention, memory, and reasoning.

Creutzfeldt-Jakob disease: A rare disease that is caused by prions that typically lead to rapid decline in memory and cognition.

Cueing: The process of providing cues, prompts, hints, and other meaningful information, direction, or instruction (such as adding labels to drawers) to assist someone with memory loss.

Deficits: Physical or cognitive skills and abilities that have been impaired or lost.

Delirium: A state of confusion, which may cause a sudden change in cognitive functioning. Delirium can have physical causes, some of which might be overlooked, such as dehydration, infection (most commonly a urinary tract infection), pneumonia, and medication.

Delusion: A false idea that is firmly believed and strongly maintained in spite of proof or evidence to the contrary.

Dementia: A term that refers to a decline in mental ability that is characterized by varying signs and symptoms such as memory loss and confusion.

Dementia umbrella: Dementia itself is an umbrella term that is used to describe various symptoms of a decline in mental ability. Alzheimer's disease, Vascular dementia, and Frontotemporal dementia are examples of different types of dementia that are categorized within the dementia umbrella.

Dementia-capable: Refers to a person who is skilled in working with individuals who have dementia and their caregivers, knowledgeable about the kinds of available services, and aware of which agencies and individuals provide such services.

Dementia-specific: Services that are provided specifically for people with dementia.

Dementia-specific care center: A facility that is solely dedicated to the care of people with dementia. This kind of facility can be free-standing or part of a larger campus.

Depression: A mood disorder that prevents a person from leading a normal life. Types of depression include major depression, bipolar depression, chronic low-grade depression (dysthymia), and seasonal depression (Seasonal Affective Disorder or SAD).

Diagnosis: The process by which a doctor or other qualified professional determines a patient's condition or disease. A diagnosis is achieved by studying the patient's symptoms, medical history, and physical or cognitive test results.

Differential diagnosis: Clinical evaluation to distinguish a condition or disease from other conditions or diseases that have similar symptoms.

Disorientation: A cognitive condition in which sense of time, direction, and spatial cognition are altered or impaired.

Durable power of attorney: A legal document that enables an individual to authorize another person, such as a trusted family member or friend, to make legal or financial decisions on their behalf if the individual becomes unable to make those decisions for him or herself.

Durable power of attorney for health care: A legal document that enables an individual to appoint another person to make health care decisions on their behalf, including choices regarding care providers, medical treatments, and end-of-life decisions.

Early-onset Alzheimer's disease: An uncommon form of Alzheimer's disease in which individuals are diagnosed before age 65. Less than 10 percent of those with Alzheimer's disease have Early-onset Alzheimer's.

Early stage: The first stages of dementia, during which an individual experiences very mild to moderate cognitive impairments.

Elder law attorney: A lawyer who practices elder law, which is a specialized area of law that focuses on issues that typically affect older adults.

Elopement: Another term for wandering.

Emotional Learning: A type of learning that occurs when a new skill is processed through the amygdala. This often occurs during life events that have emotional significance.

Experiential Learning: A type of learning that fosters focused attention through experiences. Experiential learning physically changes the brain, increases social participation, and generates multi-sensory stimulation.

Familial Alzheimer's disease: Alzheimer's disease that is hereditary (runs in families).

Frontotemporal dementia (FTD): A type of dementia that is categorized by the shrinking of the frontal and temporal anterior lobes of the brain. There are two major types of FTD: one is characterized by speech problems, the other is characterized by notable behavioral changes.

Functional capabilities: What a person is able to do.

Gait: A person's manner of walking. People in the later stages of dementia often exhibit a shuffling gait.

Glutamate: An amino acid neurotransmitter or nerve cell messenger.

Hallucination: A sense of perception (seeing, hearing, tasting, smelling, or feeling) for which no external stimulus exists.

Hippocampus: Located in the brain's limbic system, the hippocampus is where our memories are primarily stored.

Hoarding: Collecting and keeping things in a guarded manner.

Hospice: The philosophy and approach to providing comfort and care at life's end.

Huntington's disease: An inherited, degenerative brain disease that is characterized by mood changes, cognitive decline, and involuntary movement of limbs.

Incontinence: Loss of bladder or bowel control.

Instrumental activities of daily living (IADLs): Complex activities (as opposed to basic ADLs: eating, dressing and bathing) that are important to daily living, such as computing basic math, cooking, writing, and driving.

Late-onset Alzheimer's disease: The most common form of Alzheimer's disease, usually occurring after age 65. Late-onset Alzheimer's disease affects almost half of all people over the age of 85 and may or may not be hereditary.

Late stage: Designation given when dementia symptoms have progressed to the extent that a person has little capacity for self-care.

Layering: A self-securing behavior that involves unnecessarily wearing multiple layers of clothing.

Lewy body dementia (LBD): A form of dementia that is associated with protein deposits called Lewy bodies, which form in the cortex of the brain.

Living trust: A legal document that enables an individual (the grantor or trustor) to appoint someone else as trustee (usually a trusted individual or financial institution) to carefully invest and manage his or her assets.

Living Will (Advance Directive): A legal document that expresses an individual's decision regarding the use of extended care options or artificial life support systems.

Long-term care: A comprehensive range of medical, personal, and social services that are coordinated to meet the physical, social, and emotional needs of people who are chronically ill or disabled.

Long-term memory: The brain's system for permanently storing, managing, and retrieving information for later use. In healthy brains, information that is stored in long-term memory can remain there indefinitely.

Memory: The ability to process information that requires attention, storage, and retrieval.

Mild Cognitive Impairment (MCI): Refers to memory problems that are noticeable to others. People with MCI may or may not have other cognitive problems. Those with MCI alone may be able meet typical daily challenges without major difficulty. Some people with MCI progress to develop Alzheimer's disease or other forms of dementia.

Mini-Mental State Examination: A mental examination that is commonly used to measure a person's basic cognitive skills, such as short-term memory, long-term memory, spatial orientation, writing, and language.

Multi-Infarct dementia: Another term for Vascular dementia.

Neurodegenerative disease: A type of neurological disorder that is marked by the loss of nerve cells. Examples include Alzheimer's disease and Parkinson's disease.

Neurological disorder: A disturbance in the structure or function of the nervous system resulting from developmental abnormality, disease, injury, or toxin.

Neuropathology: The branch of medicine that studies nervous system diseases.

Neuroplasticity: The brain's ability to restructure its neural pathways through changes in behavior, environment, and cognitive processes such as thoughts and emotions. Plasticity refers to the brain's ability to reroute information in order to bypass damaged parts.

Neurotransmitter: A chemical that is released from a nerve cell which transmits an impulse to another nerve cell or a muscle, organ, or other tissue. A neurotransmitter transmits neurological information.

Non-pharmacological or Non-drug: Refers to a treatment approach that does not involve drugs.

Novelty learning: A type of learning that refers to learning new things, which creates new neural pathways throughout the brain that can bypass injured areas.

Onset: Defines the time when a disease begins (early-onset, late-onset).

Pacing: Aimless wandering, or walking back and forth, that is often triggered by an internal stimulus, such as pain, hunger, or boredom, or by some distraction in the environment such as an agitating noise, smell, or temperature.

Paranoia: Suspicion and mistrust of others or their actions that is not supported by evidence or justification.

Parkinson's disease: A progressive, neurodegenerative disease with an unknown cause characterized by the death of nerve cells in a specific area of the brain. People with Parkinson's disease lack the neurotransmitter dopamine and have symptoms such as tremors, speech impairments, physical difficulties, and often dementia in later stages of Parkinson's disease.

Pick's disease: A type of dementia in which abnormal amounts of certain proteins cause degeneration of nerve cells and shrinking of the brain's frontal and temporal lobes. Pick's disease causes dramatic changes in personality and social behavior but does not typically affect the memory until later stages of the disease.

Physical Learning: A type of learning that is achieved through exercise and behavioral tasks. Physical Learning can increase blood flow and foster more neural activity. Repetition of a physical action reinforces muscle memory, making physical tasks easier to perform over time.

Praxis: The ability to plan and execute coordinated movement.

Prognosis: The probable outcome or course of a disease; the estimated probability of the opportunity for recovery.

Procedural learning: Learning that is achieved through the repetition of a process or action.

Propositional knowledge: Foundational knowledge that is stored in long-term memory. This type of knowledge is governed by the hippocampus.

Pseudobulbar Affect (PBA): Occurs secondary to a variety of otherwise unrelated neurological conditions and is characterized by involuntary, sudden, and frequent episodes of laughing or crying. PBA episodes typically occur out of proportion or incongruent to the patient's underlying emotional state.

Pseudo-dementia: A person's exaggerated indifference to their environment without impairment due to cognitive capacity. Implies dementia symptoms.

Quality of care: A term that is used to rate the level of care and services. High quality care enables the recipient to attain and maintain their highest level of mental, physical, and psychological function in a dignified way.

Quality of life: A term that is used to rate a person's ability to enjoy normal life activities. Quality of life is an important consideration in medical care. Some medical treatments can seriously impair quality of life without providing appreciable benefit, while other treatments greatly enhance quality of life.

Serotonin: A natural brain chemical that affects the mood and works as a neurotransmitter.

Sensory-based learning and sensory-based knowledge: Learning that is achieved through the senses. This type of knowledge is governed by the amygdala.

Short-term memory: A system for temporarily storing and managing information that is required to carry out complex cognitive tasks such as learning, reasoning, and comprehension. Short-term memory is involved in the selection, initiation, and termination of information-processing functions such as encoding, storing, and retrieving data in the brain.

Sundowning: Unsettled behavior or increased agitation that is evident in the late afternoon, early evening, or overnight.

Trigger: Something that either sets off a disease in people who are genetically predisposed to developing the disease, or causes certain symptoms to occur in someone who has a specific disease or condition.

BIBLIOGRAPHY

"7 Stages of Alzheimer's & Symptoms | Alzheimer's
Association." Stages of Alzheimer's & Symptoms |
Alzheimer's Association. Web. 11 Nov. 2014.
<https://www.alz.org/alzheimers_disease_stages_of_
alzheimers.asp?type=alzFooter>.

"Alzheimer's Bill of Rights." Full Circle of Care Caregiver
Website. 19 Apr. 2014 <http://www.fullcirclecare.org/
alzheimers/rights.html>.

"Alzheimer's Disease Treatment: Medications and Therapies."
WebMD. WebMD, Web. 08 Sept. 2014.
<http://www.webmd.com/alzheimers/guide/treatment-
overview>.

"Alzheimer's & Dementia Weekly.": Red Plates for Eating
with Dementia. Web. 05 Dec. 2014.
<http://www.alzheimersweekly.com/2014/08/red-plates-
for-eating-with-dementia.html>.

"About Alzheimer's Foundation of America – Mission
Statement." About Alzheimer's Foundation of America –
Mission Statement. Web. 11 Oct. 2014. <http://www.
alzfdn.org/AboutUs/ missionstatement.html>.

"American Institute for Learning and Human Development:
Thomas Armstrong, Ph.D, Executive Director."
American Institute for Learning and Human
Development: Thomas Armstrong, Ph.D, Executive
Director. Web. 04 Oct. 2014. <http://institute4
learning.com/>.

"Aphasia Therapy Guide." National Aphasia Association.
Web. 15 Oct. 2014. <http://www.aphasia.org/aphasia-
resources/aphasia-therapy-guide/>.

Backer, Jos De, and Julie Sutton. The Music in Music Therapy
Psychodynamic Music Therapy in Europe: Clinical,
Theoretical and Research Approaches. London: Jessica
Kingsley, 2014. Print.

Banerjee, Sube, and Vanessa Lawrence. Managing Dementia in a Multicultural Society. Chichester, West Sussex: John Wiley & Sons, 2010. Print.

"Brain Plasticity and Alzheimer's Disease." DementiaToday. 29 Mar. 2013. Web. 23 Mar. 2015. <http://www. dementiatoday.com/brain-plasticity-and-alzheimers-disease-2/>.

Budson, Andrew E. Memory Loss, Alzheimer's Disease, and Dementia. S.l.: Elsevier - Health Science, 2015. Print.

Budson, Andrew E., and Neil W. Kowall. The Handbook of Alzheimer's Disease and Other Dementias. Chichester, West Sussex, UK: Wiley-Blackwell, 2014. Print.

Budson, Andrew E., and Paul R. Solomon. Memory Loss: A Practical Guide for Clinicians. Edinburgh?: Elsevier Saunders, 2011. Print

Bunt, Leslie, and Sarah Hoskyns. The Handbook of Music Therapy. Hove: Brunner-Routledge, 2002. Print.

"Healthy Brain Versus Alzheimer's Brain | Alzheimer's Association." Healthy Brain Versus Alzheimer's Brain | Alzheimer's Association. Web. 05 Dec. 2014. <https://www.alz.org/braintour/healthy_vs_alzheimers.asp>.

"Caregivers: Take Care of Yourselves! - HowStuffWorks." HowStuffWorks. Web. 011 Mar. 2015. <http://health.howstuffworks.com/wellness/stress-management/caregivers-take-care-of-yourselves.htm>.

"Caregiver's Guide to Understanding Dementia Behaviors." Caregiver's Guide to Understanding Dementia Behaviors. Web. 12 Mar. 2015. <https://www.caregiver.org/caregivers-guide-understanding-dementia-behaviors>.

Chapter, St. Louis. Tips for Visiting Loved Ones with Dementia. PDF. Print. 10 Jan. 2014.

Coon, Dennis, and John O. Mitterer. Psychology: A Journey. Belmont, Calif: Wadsworth/Cengage Learning, 2014. Print.

"Creating a Daily Plan | Caregiver Center | Alzheimer's Association." Alzheimer's Association. N.p., n.d. Web. 20 Sept. 2014. <http://www.alz.org/care/dementia-creating-a-plan.asp>.

"Current Treatments, Alzheimer's & Dementia | Research Center | Alzheimer's Association." Alzheimer's Association. Web. 23 Sept. 2014. <http://www.alz.org/research/science/alzheimers_disease_treatments.asp>.

"Dementia Care: What in the World Is a Dementia Village?" Alzheimers.net. 06 Aug. 2013. Web. 23 Sept. 2014. <http://www.alzheimers.net/2013-08-07/dementia-village/>.

"Dementia and Neuroplasticity: What Might Help Today – Alzheimers Disease and Other Cognitive Disorders." Dementia and Neuroplasticity: What Might Help Today – Alzheimers Disease and Other Cognitive Disorders. Web. 22 Dec. 2015. <http://www.pvmhmr.org/231-alzheimers/article/29030-dementia-and-neuroplasticity-what-might-help-today>.

"Dementia Is Not the End at CrossReach." - The Scotsman. Web. 20 Jan. 2015. <http://www.scotsman.com/news/dementia-is-not-the-end-at-crossreach-1-3550744>.

"'Dementia Village' Inspires New Care - CNN.com." CNN. Cable News Network, Web. 03 March 2015. <http://www.cnn.com/2013/07/11/world/europe/wus-holland-dementia-village/>.

"'Dementia Village' Offers Natural Alternative to Soul-crushing Nursing Homes." NaturalNews. Web. 14 Jan. 2015. <http://www.naturalnews.com/044064_Dementia_Village_Alzheimers_elderly_care.html>.

Developed By Dr. Bill Hettler, Co-Founder Of, The National Wellness Institute (Nwi), This, Interdependent Model Commonly Referred To, and As The Six Dimensions Of Wellness, Provides. The Six Dimensions of Wellness Model. PDF. Print. 01 Mar. 2015.

Doidge, Norman. Brain's Way of Healing: Remarkable Brain Recoveries and Discoveries from the Frontiers ... of Neuroplasticity. Place of Publication Not Identified: Viking, 2015. Print.

"Factsheet - Alzheimer's Association." Alxheimer's Assocation. Web. 17 May 2014 <http://www.alz.org/documents_custom/2013_facts_figures_fact_sheet.pdf_br>.

Farina, Elisabetta. Non-pharmacological Therapies in Different Types of Dementia and Mild Cognitive Impairment: A Wide Perspective from Theory to Practice. Print.

Gostick, Adrian Robert., and Chester Elton. The Carrot Principle: How the Best Managers Use Recognition to Engage Their People, Retain Talent, and Accelerate Performance. New York: Free, 2007. Print.

"Improving Alzheimer's and Dementia Care: Environmental Impact." Psych Central. Web. 10 March 2015. <http://psychcentral.com/lib/improving-alzheimers-and-dementia-care-environmental-impact/00013182>.

Kabat-Zinn, Jon. Coming to Our Senses: Healing Ourselves and the World through Mindfulness. New York: Hyperion, 2005. Print.

Kaplan, Mary, and Stephanie B. Hoffman. Behaviors in Dementia: Best Practices for Successful Management. Baltimore: Health Professions, 1998. Print.

Klerk-Rubin, Vicki De. Validation Techniques for Dementia Care: The Family Guide to Improving Communication. Baltimore: Health Professions, 2008. Print.

"Latest Alzheimer's Facts and Figures." Latest Facts & Figures Report. 17 Sept. 2013. Web. 10 Sept. 2014. <http://www.alz.org/facts/overview.asp>.

"Brain, Right Brain or Whole Brain?" Web. 4 Dec. 2014. <https://www.mindmoves.co.za/articles/article/LeftBrainRightBrainOrWholeBrain.pdf>.

Lipton, Anne M., and Cindy D. Marshall. The Common Sense Guide to Dementia for Clinicians and Caregivers. New York, NY: Springer, 2013. Print.

Luminet, Olivier, and Antonietta Curci. Flashbulb Memories: New Issues and New Perspectives. Hove (UK): Psychology, 2009. Print.

Luthra, Atul Sunny. The Meaning of Behaviors in
    Dementia/neurocognitive Disorders: New Terminology,
    Classification, and Behavioral Management. N.p.: n.p.,
    n.d. Print.

Mace, Nancy L., and Peter V. Rabins. The 36-hour Day: A
    Family Guide to Caring for People Who Have Alzheimer
    Disease, Related Dementias, and Memory Loss.
    Baltimore: Johns Hopkins UP, 2011. Print

Mahoney, Ellen, Ladislav Volicer, and Ann Hurley.
    Management of Challenging Behaviors in Dementia.
    Baltimore: Health Professions, 2000. Print.

"The Brain–Heart Connection." The Brain–Heart Connection.
    Web. 05 Oct. 20154.
    <http://circ.ahajournals.org/content/116/1/77.extract>.

Meadows, Anthony. Developments in Music Therapy
    Practice: Case Study Perspectives. Gilsum, NH:
    Barcelona, 2011. Print.

"Memory Loss Myths & Facts | Alzheimer's Association."
    Memory Loss Myths & Facts | Alzheimer's Association.
    Web. 05 Oct. 2014.
    <http://www.alz.org/alzheimers_disease_myths_about_
    alzheimers.asp>.

"Music Therapy in Dementia Treatment - Recollection
    Through Sound." Music Therapy in Dementia Treatment.
    Web. 10 Nov. 2014.
    <http://www.todaysgeriatricmedicine.com/news/
    story1.shtml>.

"Myths and Realities about Alzheimer's Disease." Myths and
    Realities about Alzheimer's Disease. Web. 10
    Feb. 2015. <http://www.alzheimer.ca/en/About-
    dementia/Alzheimer-s-disease/Myth-and-reality-about-
    Alzheimer-s-disease>.

"Policy Brief: The Global Impact of Dementia 2013-2050."
    Policy Brief: The Global Impact of Dementia 2013-2050.
    Web. 15 Oct. 2014.
    <http://www.alz.co.uk/research/G8-policy-brief>.

"Residential Care | Caregiver Center | Alzheimer's Association." Alzheimer's Association. Web. 14 Oct. 2014. <http://www.alz.org/care/alzheimers-dementia-residential-facilities.asp>.

Sacks, Oliver W. Musicophilia: Tales of Music and the Brain. New York: Alfred A. Knopf, 2007. Print.

Shannon, Joyce Brennfleck. Brain Disorders Sourcebook: Basic Consumer Health Information about Acquired and Traumatic Brain Injuries, Brain Tumors, Cerebral Palsy and Other Genetic and Congenital Brain Disorders, Infections of the Brain, Epilepsy, and Degenerative Neurological Disorders Such as Dementia, Huntington Disease, and Amyotrophic Lateral Sclerosis (ALS): Along with Information on Brain Structure and Function, Treatment and Rehabilitation Options, a Glossary of Terms Related to Brain Disorders, and a Directory of Resources for More Information. Detroit, MI: Omnigraphics, 2010. Print.

Siegel, Daniel J. Mindsight: The New Science of Personal Transformation. New York: Bantam, 2010. Print.

Smart, Colette M. "Mindfulness Training: A Novel Approach to Intervening in Older Adults with Subjective Cognitive Decline." Alzheimer's & Dementia 10.4 (2014): P164. Web.

Smith, Glenn E., and Mark W. Bondi. Mild Cognitive Impairment and Dementia: Definitions, Diagnosis, and Treatment. New York: Oxford UP, 2013. Print.

"The 3 R's of Habit Change: How To Start New Habits That Actually Stick." Web. 11 Dec. 2014. <http://jamesclear.com/three-steps-habit-change>.

"The Stages Of Dementia." The Stages of Dementia. Web. 10 Sept. 2014. <http://www.dementia.org/symptoms/stages-of-dementia>.

"Stages and Behaviors | Caregiver Center | Alzheimer's Association." Alzheimer's Association. Web. 14 Oct. 2014. <http://www.alz.org/care/alzheimers-dementia-stages-behaviors.asp>.

"The Art of the Compliment." Psychology Today.
     Web. 03 Jan. 2015.
     <https://www.psychologytoday.com/articles/200403/the
     art-the-compliment>.
"Until There Is a Cure: Non-Pharmacological Approaches to
     Dementia Care | Alz.org/nyc." Until There Is a Cure:
     Non-Pharmacological Approaches to Dementia Care |
     Alz.org/nyc. Web. 22 Oct. 2014.
     <http://www.alznyc.org/nyc/newsletter/summer2012/
     02.asp#.VUgoA2ctDIU>.
"Understanding Dementia." : Signs, Symptoms, Types, and
     Treatment. Web. 10 Dec. 2014.
     <http://www.helpguide.org/articles/alzheimers-
     dementia/understanding-dementia.htm>.
"Understanding Validation: A Way to Communicate
     Acceptance." Psychology Today. Web. 06 Nov.
     2014. <https://www.psychologytoday.com/blog/pieces-
     mind/201204/understanding-validation-way-
     communicate-acceptance>.
"What Is Dementia?" Dementia – Signs, Symptoms, Causes,
     Tests, Treatment, Care. Web. 12 Nov. 2014.
     <http://www.alz.org/what-is-dementia.asp>.
"Why a Daily Routine Is Helpful for People with Dementia."
     AgingCare. Web. 04 Feb. 2015.
     <http://www.agingcare.com/Articles/daily-routine-for-
     people-with-dementia-156855.htm>.
Wimo, Anders, and Martin Prince. World Alzheimer Report
     2010 the Global Economic Impact of Dementia. London,
     UK: Alzheimer's Disease International, 2010. Print.

Made in the USA
Middletown, DE
07 November 2015